Triumphing Over Cancer

David's Miracle Story

Plus

Forty Survival Strategies You Can Use

Dr. Judith Rolfs

Triumphing Over Cancer

Copyright

Medical Disclaimer

The information in this book is not intended or implied
to be a substitute for professional medical advice,
diagnosis or treatment. The author assumes no
responsibility or liability for any losses or damages
arising from any information within this book. The ideas,
techniques and suggestions are for informational
purposes only and are not a substitute for consultation
with a professional health care provider. We
recommend a combination of the best medical,
emotional and spiritual treatment available.

WHAT READERS ARE SAYING:

"This story has got to be heard today! I stayed up all night to read... Once I started I couldn't stop."

Joann McLuen,
Director of Women's Programs,
Colbert, Georgia

"What a blessing! As I pondered the Lord reminded me that my family was experiencing a long-drawn out trial, too and that I could have hope for a magnificent healing also. It was then that I realized that this book belongs in the hands of anyone experiencing a difficult or 'hopeless' situation (And that's most folks!)"

Kathy Majka, Orlando, FL

"Just finished and had to write to tell you it's wonderful...in the true sense of the word, it's wonder-full. Full of the wonder of faith in the face of all the horrors you all had to deal with. I thrill at the thoughts of how many will be helped by your sharing."

Sue Drefs, Delavan, WI

"Your book leaves me speechless. I cried the first four chapters, then was captivated and amazed by your ability to react so intellectually, yet spiritually during such an emotional and physically draining episode of your life. I feel as though I am magnetically drawn to you through your writing. I am hooked, and desire to read everything you've ever written."

Marianne Mortenson, IL

"I appreciated your sharing your inspiring book. Many messages gave me insight and I shall in the future reflect on them. I appreciated the book because at the time of diagnosis one is very confused and upset and looking for the right path to cope with what is ahead."

Marcia Baldree

"*Triumphing Over Cancer* was not merely inspiring, but full of practical advice... I keep it close at hand as a reference book."

Cynthia Rauland, Walworth, WI

DEDICATION

This is your story David and the story of others who face a life-threatening illness. When times are tough in the future as they will be occasionally, may you always remember God is a real and present help in trouble and His people are all over the world. Most amazing of all, when earthly help is exhausted, God often sends angels into your midst, as He did for you.

PREFACE

Dear Reader,

When a life-threatening illness hits, you aren't prepared. There's more than one way to attack a monster like cancer. You need to get yourself briefed on all the ways that work!

Healing is a combination of spiritual, physical, and emotional factors - each of us is composed of body, mind and spirit.

Doctors have their place, but it's easy to forget God, when you feel quite comfortable with your doctor's expertise and skill. That's not God's plan. Use doctors appropriately, but also put your faith in God.

Has illness led you or your loved one to a faith crisis? Are you bouncing around spiritually wondering if all this God stuff is real? How far can you trust God? What is your part as a patient or caregiver? Are your thoughts clear about what you believe?

God never said there'd be no pain in this world, but He did say there'd be a way around it or through it. We live among ugly things like sin and sickness. Struggling against them is a physical and spiritual battle. The grace and the wisdom for the fight come from God.

When the smooth way gets rough, when all the plans go awry, what's happening then? Has God deserted you and moved on to help someone else? It may be tempting to think that, but it's not true!

There may be mistakes during diagnostic testing and treatment that could have been avoided. Family members and friends, too, have said and done things that are hurtful. It's hard to forgive, but essential. This whole life experience is about accepting imperfect people and circumstances. We live on earth not in heaven.

It's important to focus on the joy that's visible each day in simple ways. The kind gesture of a friend; the softness of a smooth fabric; the tree in your yard you hadn't noticed lately. You're here - alive - in this moment safe - and with God who loves you. Jesus is as real as the sun. Joy!

First it seems unbearable. Why this horrible illness? For learning to value life and God and other people? For learning to appreciate more? Whatever, God knows, He cares and is at work.

Not everybody is going to agree with the treatment choices you need to make. Some people will think you're crazy for thinking that God cares and that God is going to get involved in your situation. Tune out the people that bring you and your loved one down.

Some day no more death! Revelation 21: 3 and 4 reads: "I heard a loud voice from the throne saying, 'Now the dwelling of God is with men, and He will live with them. They will be His people, and God Himself will be with them and be their God. He will wipe every tear from their eyes. There will be no more death or mourning or crying or pain, for the old order of things has passed away." (NIV) That's what's ahead. But until then, you've got to hold the ground here and now. May this true story and the principles in *Triumphing Over Cancer* which is a patient and caregiver's journey help you achieve victory.

CHAPTER 1

David. God's gentle son, spirit of laughter; essence of craziness. How we loved him!

As we walked to our brown Chrysler in the hospital parking lot feeling the harsh chill of the bitter air and the lingering, horrifying words of the emergency room doctor, we were frozen in private worlds of shock. The sounds of my footsteps slapping against the pavement seemed to echo in my ears, "Cancer. Cancer. Life-must-never-be-taken-for-granted."

Twenty minutes ago in the emergency examining room David was silent. Now he spouted. "I knew something was very wrong, I kept telling the doctors. Now I've got a death bomb in my body. Cancer!"

Disgustedly David folded his handsome five-foot-ten inch frame into the dark privacy of the back seat. In a forlorn tone he continued, "It's not that I'm afraid to die. I believe that I'll be with God, but I'm not ready yet!" David coughed away a choked sob.

Thank God darkness hid the tears streaming down my own cheeks. Glancing into the rear-view mirror, I spoke to David's reflection huddled in the corner. "We know it's scary, son, we know, but we're going to fight this." I hoped my voice was encouraging.

After another long silence, David said, "Mom, I don't want any of my friends to know."

"You're not ashamed or embarrassed I hope! This isn't your fault." Did David see cancer as a blight on his emergent male image?

"David, if anyone is responsible perhaps it's me-- something I did or didn't do for your diet or whatever." My motherly thoughts were flying around irrationally too.

"Son, there's a couple of our friends I want to tell so they can pray," Wayne said. "I'll ask them to keep it quiet, if you like."

"Okay," came David's subdued response.

Pulling into our driveway, I was struck by the total aura of unreality. How could our cozy, hundred-year-old Victorian house be sitting as we'd left it that afternoon with the comforting sound of lake water lapping at the beach? Dear God, let me wake up from this monstrous dream! I pleaded silently while I wanted to yell, God, where have you been? Come now to protect him.

Not since David was a young child had Wayne and I both tucked him into bed. Maybe reliving times past could turn back the family clock and erase the ugly present. I knew better, but I was operating on my feelings.

Wayne's "Try not to worry, David" was obviously a waste of words. Fortunately. Dr. Naraldi had given David a sedative for sleep.

There was little sleep for Wayne or I that night.

I closed the family room door behind me, wanting to be alone with the Lord. God, I'm not even going to ask, Why David, he's so good? I know no one is privileged to avoid all sickness and suffering. As a professional counselor I'd helped other families deal with the pain of life-threatening illness. Being emotionally involved now made it hard to be objective.

Lord, we need to know what to do. Prayer? Lord, how do we really pray? How do we pray for something as big as life itself? How is your healing released today?

I wanted answers. I wished with all my heart that Jesus still walked the earth and talked audibly.

Soon Wayne came in and slumped onto the sofa seat next to me. "Where did we go wrong?" I moaned and collapsed into his arms.

4

Wayne reiterated my agonized feelings. "I feel as if my heart just broke," he said with anguish.

"I blame myself," I said. "In my eagerness for David to be well, I'd assumed the doctors were correct with their simple explanations for his symptoms. Perhaps if I'd looked more closely I might have seen signs that the doctors were missing."

"If onlys" bombarded me.

Wayne stopped me. "When Jesus healed the paralyzed man his disciples wanted to know if it was the man's own sins or the sins of his parents that had caused his illness. Jesus' answer was neither. 'But only that the glory of God might be made manifest.' That needs to be our focus too! God blessed us with children. We have to trust that He knows what is happening now, and is at work."

I thought about David and his sisters, Tamara, 22, Pamela, 21, and his brother, Dan, 13. Our delight in them spilled over into their relationships with one another making our family bond strong physically and emotionally. I cried afresh thinking how devastated his sisters and brother would be when we told them. I closed my eyes and prayed aloud:

"Eighteen years old.

It wouldn't be right, God.

David's grown from an impulsive, delightful child to a strong-willed, enthusiastic man.

His long awaited time, 'When you grow up' has come. The time to live his dreams has just begun.

Don't let it end like this.

Cancer, be gone!"

Wayne added, "Amen. It's going to take time and grace to work through our feelings. First how do we lift this heavy stupor of shock so we can function?"

About 2 a.m. Wayne and I still hadn't moved from the family room sofa. We had our arms around each other. I was crying softly. I looked out the picture window through my tears and saw a foot-long, radiant light outside. Rays projected brightly in every direction. I thought it was probably the streetlight. Or was it?

As we talked, I kept my head steady so that my eyes could watch the light. It was strangely comforting. The light seemed to me to be David's life. Suddenly the light was no longer visible. I panicked. After a few seconds it came back, then went out and came back on again. This happened twice. I sensed this was a sign from Our Lord that David would come very close to death twice but he would come back.

I had never had an actual sign from the Lord before. If anyone asked me how I knew this was one, I couldn't say, but I knew. I remembered this moment many times over in the coming months.

CHAPTER 2

Exhausted, but hopeful I went to bed. Before I could fall asleep the events of summer tumbled through my mind.

The first outward sign of trouble began in June 1985, just after David's eighteenth birthday. The beginning was pain. What a falsely simple, four-letter word!

"Hey guys, I've got this pain in my right shoulder blade. I feel knocked out by it." At work at the golf pro shop as a bag boy, David became shaky and nauseous. "I'm going to the back room to rest."

David's fellow workers teased him. "What a wimp! Out too late, huh, Dave?"

David, too exhausted to care, ignored them. Then came a parade of discomfort: jaw pain, leg pain, and chest pain.

"Mom, everything hurts!" David said to me one night in early August. With each new series of pains David went to the doctor. Not just once. At least ten times he visited doctors in various specialties and was continually misdiagnosed.

"Mrs. Rolfs," our family doctor's tone was reassuring, "this pain in David's back is from his job at the golf course. He's pulled a muscle carrying heavy bags of clubs. Nothing to worry about."

He handed David a prescription. "Get this muscle relaxant. Take it easy for a few weeks. You'll be good as new." But the pain didn't stop. Members of our extended family encouraged David with marvelous anecdotes of helpful chiropractic treatment. David dutifully began visits to a chiropractor three times a week.

"I'm sure, David, that your back pain is the consequence of a misaligned spine," the chiropractor said confidently. "I can correct that with several weeks of treatment."

"Okay, doctor, crack my back, and stop the pain." But the pain remained.

Then David's nocturnal mouth pain started. "Mom, I've got this pain way back in my jawbone. It's waking me up at night with pain that lasts for hours."

"I'll make a dentist appointment for you - perhaps your wisdom teeth are the problem." David's dad and our daughter, Tamara, had needed surgical removal of wisdom teeth.

A visit to the dentist confirmed this suspicion - impacted wisdom teeth. I asked for a second opinion from an oral surgeon. He said, "David's wisdom teeth are not infected It's unusual, but not impossible, for him to have as much pain as he's described. We better take the teeth out just the same."

Out they came, but the pain continued to flare up off and on and so did a low grade fever.

David had faith in us. We put our faith in medical knowledge, but the circle of pain never stopped. It just grew wider. I began to wonder if David had a serious illness. I had lost a first cousin at the age of eighteen to bone cancer, but there was no similarity between their symptoms. I put the thought out of my mind. Two weeks after the oral surgery, David still had pain and a low-grade fever.

After repeated calls and return visits to the oral surgeon, I got the subtle impression David was viewed as a hypochondriac by the doctor's receptionist and nurse. On our last visit, we were told, "We're observing David as a surgical case with rare complications." Alarm bells began to sound inside me in light of David's other symptoms.

8

Simultaneously, David developed severe leg pain. Since he'd done some running in high school, two different doctors concluded he had shin splints.

What next, Lord? We were totally perplexed.

"Wrap his legs tightly each day," our family doctor recommended matter-of-factly. Eventually the pain will go away. Take this prescription of aspirin with codeine for severe pain." David walked with wraps on his legs to alleviate shin splint pain. Logical again, and again very wrong.

Each day we prayed for David's healing from these troublesome problems. In the meantime, David appeared to be losing weight. But who wouldn't after the liquid, then soft diet following oral surgery and all the pain and loss of sleep he endured?

Despite David's symptoms, the simple, natural medical explanations appeased us. True, many problems had cropped up at once, but they were coincidental, the doctors said. In between, David had brief spells of pain free normality.

In mid-August, David excitedly headed off to college at the University of Wisconsin-Whitewater. He immediately joined a parachute-jumping club and received an assignment as a reporter on the college cable television station. Although David had no acting experience, he tried out for a part in his college's presentation of Cabaret. Energetic David thought he could do anything if he tried hard enough -- one of the last of the Horatio Algiers. Until, that is, until…

During these three months, David was medicated by his various doctors with muscle relaxants, aspirin with codeine, and antibiotics. Often he moved in a misty haze of reality.

A friend said, "Perhaps David needs to toughen up a bit. He probably has a low threshold for pain."

Wayne and I couldn't accept that. Surely this was just a run of misfortune. All these clues implied something was seriously wrong, but the doctors scoffed at our concern.

At the end of August David came home to be an usher in his sister's wedding. He awoke during the night with such tremendous pain in his jaw and legs that he couldn't sleep. I was surprised at the increased severity of his pain.

The morning of our daughter's wedding I said to the rest of the family, "Wedding or not, I'm taking David to the oral surgeon and internist. Something's not right!"

I told our doctor, "My daughter is getting married in a couple hours. I wouldn't be here this morning if I wasn't extremely concerned." I said the word for the first time. "Doctor please check my son for cancer," even though I hated saying the word in front of David. "I don't understand what's happening to him."

The doctor performed a test on David's legs, an electrolyte test, which came back negative. Again we were reassured David would be fine.

Later, I learned this definitely was not the appropriate test. If any doctor had done a simple white blood count they would have seen that David's white blood cells were reproducing out-of-control. Through procedural slip-ups, the nurse at the M.D.'s office had neglected to take his blood pressure on his two previous visits. It had skyrocketed.

Again David received heavy-duty pain medication.

Just before the wedding guests arrived, David stood in the center aisle of church surrounded by a group of Christian young men who prayed for his healing — a scene that was to be repeated countless times in the months ahead. David managed to get through the wedding ceremony, but totally missed the reception. He went home and slept by the mercy of pain medication for twenty hours straight.

After the August wedding weekend, David returned to college and continued to have intermittent, severe pains. Life was endurable for him only with the more than ten bottles of antibiotics, pain pills, sleeping pills, and muscle relaxants he'd been given.

We next saw David the third weekend in September. When he arrived Friday night, he was hunched to one side because of chest pain that occurred when he had tried running on the college track. He hastily unpacked his bag and shoved it into a drawer.

"I just want to go to bed."

"David, let me take you to the doctor right now."

He answered angrily, "Mom, all my past visits haven't brought me any relief."

I was annoyed with David; I still thought medical treatment could help.

"I'll go tomorrow, I need sleep now!"

The next day David kept his previously scheduled appointment with the chiropractor. I insisted on going along.

The chiropractor spoke sympathetically and claimed, "David's doing lots better, Mrs. Rolfs. This new pain in his chest is only a secondary result of the healing that's occurring as David's spine moves into alignment."

I believed him. I didn't know he hadn't ex-rayed David's chest -only his spinal column.

The next day, after enduring four months of continual pain, a correct diagnosis was finally made. At about 9:00 p.m. we were returning from a trip to Illinois to celebrate David's Grandpa's 75th birthday. From the back seat of the car, David said disgustedly. "Great! Now my scalp is bothering me. I must be reacting to this new shampoo I've been using."

David asked me to feel his head. I reached back. Beneath his thick brown hair, my hand rested upon nickel-sized lumps. About a dozen had popped out all over his head.

I flinched in horror because I knew beyond a shadow of doubt that something terrible was wrong with my son.

In a voice that echoed throughout the car with its unnaturally high pitch, I said to Wayne, "We can't go home. We need to take David immediately to the nearest hospital emergency room."

Even in the darkness, I could feel my husband's glance of amazement. He started to voice a reasonable objection, and then stopped and turned the car around. Within ten minutes we saw signs for Humana Hospital in Hoffman Estates, Illinois. How fortunate that we were so close --the first of many such happenings in the year ahead.

Since David looked fine, I imagine the three of us were a strange sight walking into that emergency room. The receptionist looked up with a queer expression when I said, "Our son has bumps on his head." Obviously David hadn't fallen off his tricycle and since he was bigger than either of us, he wasn't an abused child.

"Age?" she asked.

"Eighteen."

"How did he get them? Was there an accident?"

I answered impatiently, "We don't know."

I ignored her gaze because I couldn't care less what she or anyone else thought. I'd become a mother tiger fighting for my cub. "We also want the pain in his chest examined," I added.

About an hour and two x-rays later, the entire staff became very solicitous. Dr. Naraldi called us outside of David's room as he slapped the x-rays on the hallway-viewing screen.

In a whispery voice the doctor told us what he suspected. "See the large mediastinal chest mass. That's interfering with his breathing; the lumps on his head are a confirmation -– a problem with the lymph system." Dr. Naraldi was a young doctor, and it was hard for him to get the words out.

"What are you saying, doctor?" Wayne demanded.

The doctor spoke gently. "We can't be certain without a biopsy, of course, but the signs strongly indicate cancer." Somehow we knew it already from his face, but we had to hear the word to believe it.

I couldn't swallow. I tried to retreat to the blissful state of denial. David was young and healthy. It couldn't be! But I knew deep inside I'd finally heard the dreaded truth.

The word resounded ceaselessly or was it my head that was going round and round. A large tumor in his chest and cancerous nodules on his head. No wonder David had trouble running around the college track! Dear God, David tried to live normally. We knew he'd been ill. Ill, but not sick to death.

I noticed David peering through the examining room door. He looked like a frightened deer. Obviously the tone of our voices outside his room alarmed him. I turned and said to the doctor, "We need to tell David."

We reentered the room. A long silence followed as we waited for the doctor to speak again. He began with vague, technical terms and obviously struggled with the words, which only increased David's anxiety.

I heard myself interrupting, "David, the doctor thinks you have cancer. As bad as that may sound, nowadays there are incredible treatments and cures. You are going to be alright." A positive initial response to this devastating news was essential, I realized instinctively.

Young Dr. Naraldi recovered his control. I wondered if he'd ever given this news to anyone before. He seemed very moved. "You need to begin treatment immediately —

tomorrow. I suggest Madison, a major cancer center that's fortunately close to your home in Wisconsin."

David's eyes darted back and forth as though pleading, say this isn't true. His colorless face expressed clearly that he knew he'd heard his potential death sentence. He said nothing further.

"We'll prepare a file with your ex-rays to take with you."

Wayne nodded, still unable to speak.

I said, "We're in this with you all the way son. We'll do whatever it takes to get you well." Reassuring, confident words let them be true, Lord!

As we waited for David's records, my thoughts raged out of control. Our precious son! I wanted to wrap him up in my arms and take him away. But there was no safe place, because he now carried his own enemy within! Oh dear God – how could this happen?

At the same time I was furious. For four months we'd believed the doctors' comforting explanations of pulled muscles, shin splints, infected wisdom teeth. I relived the memory of trying to support David as he staggered to the car still groggy from the anesthetic of oral surgery. I remembered him as he looked propped on the sofa, holding ice bags on his swollen cheeks after the surgery.

The chiropractor only the day before had claimed David was getting better. He had sounded knowledgeable and we wanted desperately to believe him. On September 24, 1985 at Humana Hospital, Doctor Naraldi had ordered the right tests and revealed the devastating truth.

I knew I needed to surrender my anger and control the cold fear. Instead I wanted to pass out right where I stood, and find out this was unreal, a dream. I couldn't stop my runaway emotions.

David's birth flashed through my mind. We almost lost him during delivery due to RH blood factor

14

complications and a placenta previa condition. Now this! A whirlwind surged through my spinning mind.

I caught Wayne's eye and looked at his shocked, silent face, the mirror of my own pain. Our emotional distress didn't matter. How could we best help David? We certainly hadn't done well enough prior to this night.

We couldn't waste energy on what used to be or could have been. I told myself not to think now about Dave's carefree youth. It's over. He's no longer one of the guys. This ugly cursed cancer would separate him in ways we could only guess.

A bolt of something, grace is the only word, helped me pull myself together.

Vague symptoms no longer hid the horrible truth. There was a slight surge of emotion at having identified the enemy at last. Dear God, what existed was cancer, and we had to stop it.

CHAPTER 3

Morning came at last and with it a sense of urgency. Nothing mattered except getting this cancer out of David. I called a friend, whose daughter had been treated for Hodgkin's disease, and questioned her. Concern and tenderness flowed from her voice as she recommended her daughter's doctor.

After we made an 11 a.m. appointment at a clinic in Madison, Wisconsin we began to feel a little better. I assumed doctors knew a lot about healing cancer; I hoped it was enough. Does anyone know enough yet?

Suddenly, from perhaps the nudge of the Spirit, a reminder came to us. We were in the process of changing our health insurance to another company. I couldn't care less about finances. I thought, take our house, our money, whatever for the life of our son. Still we had to be certain we could provide the treatment David needed.

Wayne called and renewed our insurance with our present company because the new one might reject us now. The deadline for renewal had almost expired, a visible instance of God's incredible timing. Then we headed for Madison.

An hour and a half later we pulled up to a small clinic, an unimpressive, squat little building. Somehow I imagined that a place where people were healed of cancer should look like a massive walled fortress.

As we apprehensively walked into a tiny consulting room, a young doctor with a shock of brown hair appeared. We gave him our file, and waited while he went to another room to examine the x-rays.

His face was emotionally unchanged when he returned.

Speaking directly to David, he said matter-of-factly, "I concur with the preliminary diagnosis of cancer of the lymph system, David. We need a biopsy to determine if this is Hodgkin's or another form of lymphoma. The treatment procedure we follow depends on the exact type of cancer. Also we'll do a spinal tap and a bone marrow test tomorrow to see if the cancer has spread to your nervous system or bone marrow." He sounded like a mechanic explaining a car repair.

I gave an involuntary gasp. "You mean there could be even more?"

"We'll know after the tests."

David asked, "How long will this take? I'm a college freshman, I can't miss too many classes."

The doctor looked up surprised. School didn't rate like the treatment schedule, but he realized it was significant to David. "We'll try to work around your class schedule, but I can't guarantee we always can."

Then David asked the big question that concerned us most, "What are my chances?"

The doctor replied in a steady voice, "David, if your biopsy confirms what we suspect, I'd estimate that you have a 50-50 chance of survival with intense radiation and chemotherapy treatments. There will be some side effects like lose of your hair, and perhaps, but not always, loss of reproductive function."

David's body went limp.

Blunt words. Was there a gentler way? Might more hope have been offered like someone's got to be in the 50% that survives? It might as well be you.

The doctor's low-key manner gave the impression that he wasn't highly optimistic. I had studied enough research reports about the immune system to know the importance of positive attitude. The doctor's blasé manner irritated me.

Where is our twentieth century medical expertise? I thought. "50-50 odds are the best we have?" I blurted out. Odds! Like a horse race. The stark reality of these statistics shattered us. *My God, my God do not forsake us. We need you desperately,* I prayed silently. Medical science doesn't offer enough hope.

We made an appointment for that afternoon with Dr. Burnhardt, a surgeon, to discuss the biopsy.

On the way out, we asked a pink-garbed receptionist if there was another treatment center in Madison. We wanted a second opinion.

"Yeah, the University of Wisconsin-Madison Hospital has a cancer clinic."

We called and a compassionate receptionist squeezed us in for an appointment after lunch.

Outside David contemplated his future. "Losing my hair, perhaps losing my ability to have children. I'm not sure it's worth living like that ... " his voice trailed off.

"It's tough, Son, but your hair will grow back and you can always adopt children." Wayne tried to sound comforting.

David retorted angrily, "I don't want to adopt, I want my own kids!"

"C'mon, let's get some lunch," Wayne said softly.

Over sandwiches that we scarcely ate, David commented wryly, "It would have helped if I'd ever won a contest or a raffle in my life. It's hard for me to picture myself on the winning side."

"David, you can be," I assured him, using positive words, but what did we know about how to help. It took us four months to get a correct diagnosis!

Our ignorance about cancer was appalling. We needed more information and we had to get it fast. With all the diseases in the world what parent can ever be prepared for the tragedy that can strike our children?

18

I prayed aloud, "Lord, give us your wisdom."

After lunch, we got lost going over to the University but it didn't matter that we were late. The doctors were hours behind schedule.

Nothing in our lives had prepared us for our first sight of a major hospital's cancer clinic waiting room. Outpatients arrived with facemasks covering their noses and mouths. Shiny bald-headed men and women wearing scarves over hairless scalps paced the adjoining corridors. Most kept their eyes downcast discouraging conversation. Those with masks kept a careful distance from the others.

At first, I thought the patients were contagious. I soon learned masks were intended to protect those with low immune function from the germs of others. Chemotherapy lowers the body's white blood cell count critical for fighting germs. Usually after treatment the count is naturally restored over a few days to weeks of time.

In the meantime, extreme precaution against germs is necessary. A patient can die, not from cancer, but from the side effects of the treatment being used as a cure. Cancer treatment is radiation, chemotherapy, surgery. Burn it, poison it, rip it out. No illness on the face of the earth is treated as radically.

I whispered to Wayne, "Surely this disease is the scourge of hell itself. My heart wants to whisk David away." I forced myself to sit down to wait our turn. There was little, if any, chitchat among the patients. Some hid in magazine reading. I sat quietly praying for David and for these other afflicted patients as well.

Time passed dreadfully slowly for the next hour and a half. We watched doctors and nurses enter examination rooms that bordered a long central corridor. Each time they emerged we hoped futilely that our time had come. Disappointed, we finally had to leave or miss the 4 p.m. appointment with the surgeon back at the smaller clinic.

Months later we understood the difficulty of scheduling these appointments and realized why there can be so many delays. The doctors don't know in advance what procedures each patient might require because their condition can change so quickly. All of these people are fighting to stay alive; every moment is precious. Cancer is a horrible disease, a thief. It robs its victims of the short time they have to love one another on earth.

Our meeting with the surgeon, a kindly looking fiftyish doctor, gave us our first hope.

"David, you're young, you have an excellent chance of beating this. I'll fit you in for a biopsy tomorrow first thing before my other surgeries. Otherwise, you'd have to wait three days because my schedule is full. You'll have to be here by 5:30 a.m. though. The sooner we get that biopsy, the sooner you can begin treatment and lick this!"

Dr. Burnhardt turned toward us. "Don't you worry, I'll treat David as though he were my own son."

We felt as though a sheet of kindness dropped mercifully.

There seemed to be little doubt about the general diagnosis, but this biopsy would provide essential information about cancer type. We stopped back at the oncologist's office. We were assured that David would receive the same treatment as at the University Clinic, where his oncologist had been a former staff member.

We agreed to proceed with the program he recommended after getting a second opinion about the protocol from Mayo Clinic.

As we waited in the pharmacy for a prednisone prescription, I described my "sign of light" to David.

David asked, "How can you be sure this was a sign from God?" His voice mingled hope with skepticism.

I said, "I just know. If I wanted to dream something up, I would never have you come close to death twice."

"True." David sighed. "I hope you're right Mom."

The three of us trudged back to our car, and drove home feeling as though we'd walked the eighty miles back.

CHAPTER 4

At daybreak we were on our way to St. Mary's Hospital in Madison. Before the biopsy, the surgeon stopped in to see us.

David said, "I don't want to have scars all over my body."

I could guess Dr. Burnhardt's thoughts. *We're trying to save your life and you're concerned about one-inch scars!*

Dr. Burnhardt reassured David, "I'll do my best to keep them small." He explained where he'd make the incisions on David's chest and head.

Before David was wheeled off to surgery, Wayne and I prayed with him, "Heavenly Father, he's your son as well as ours, dedicated to you, keep him safe. Jesus, watch over this procedure and use it as a step toward his recovery. In your name we pray. Amen."

Waiting with anticipation in David's empty hospital room, we heard a familiar, booming "Hi," from our good friend Bob Drefs.

"Bob, what are you doing here?" Wayne exclaimed.

"I planned my work schedule to include Madison calls so I could be here during the biopsy. How's it going?"

We filled him in briefly, fighting back tears.

Bob confided, "I'm organizing an evening of prayer. We've got to get some prayer power going on this."

"Thanks!" Wayne said gratefully.

Intercessory prayer, I thought, *Lord, yes, I believe in its power. Sometimes it seems to work, sometimes it doesn't. Why Lord? Is it numbers, consistency? Teach me.*

About an hour later, David was wheeled back into his room, still groggy, but alert. Dr. Burnhardt reported that the surgery went well. "The incisions are as unobtrusive as possible. I think David will be pleased."

"Thanks, doctor." I took a deep breath.

"Preliminary pathology confirms the diagnosis. Remember he's young, I believe he can beat this! Good luck." With that the surgeon left.

"Lord, there's no doubt now, get those ugly cancer cells out of his body!" Wayne and I prayed.

The considerate head nurse came into David's room to ask us, "How are you holding up?"

"We're doing okay but then, what is okay anymore?" I asked sadly. "David's our big concern."

She agreed, but added, "If you don't take care of yourselves, you won't be able to meet his needs." The nurse suggested tranquilizers for me temporarily.

I refused. Whatever there was to know and feel, I want to be fully alert. David, Wayne and I had to think clearly for the decisions ahead. There couldn't be any more mistakes.

The oncologist arrived. "I need to do a spinal tap and bone marrow test before David can leave. Would you like to wait in the hall or watch?"

"We'll stay," we said unison. We didn't want to observe but had to keep a protective eye upon every procedure. This was our son's body being invaded.

The doctor told David, 'You need to roll onto your stomach." After swabbing a four by four inch area, he injected an anesthetic, then a long needle, explaining as he worked. "This will remove a small amount of fluid from your spinal column to be tested for cancer cells." An assistant stood by ready to rush the specimens to the lab immediately.

The bone marrow test was even worse. "David, bones aren't hard and brittle within the body, as most people think. They're tough and almost rubbery in texture especially in younger patients like you. We need to remove an actual particle from within the bone, but first we must penetrate it. Sometimes we can extract it on the first try, other times, we must go in over and over until we have a usable specimen." Extracting his instrument, the doctor remarked, "This will work."

"Thank God," I said quietly. "The doctor got it the first time." *God, is this how you felt watching the nails penetrate Your Son's skin?*

The oncologist asked David, "How was it?"

"It felt like you were grinding your way through my hip, then I felt a sharp shot of pain when you pierced the bone."

Oh Lord! How I wished I could be on the table instead of him!

In the late afternoon, weak and still groggy, David was released from the hospital. He'd been watching the clock. "Dad. I can still make my driver's class in Elkhorn."

"If you're sure you're up to it, we'll take you," Wayne said, "Yes," David answered determinedly.

During the sleepless nights, nocturnal sweats and drugged days of this last summer David had a tough time making it to work at 6 a.m. Twice after oversleeping he got a speeding ticket hurrying to work. This special driver education class would wipe out adverse points on his driving record.

We drove directly to David's class from his biopsy surgery, getting a hamburger along the way. David walked in, bandages and all. He - we - had an unspoken pact.

We'd never stop living fully in the present, while we fought for the future.

After we dropped David off. I couldn't hold back the anguish I was feeling. Wayne pulled off on a quiet county road and held me. We cried together.

"Instead of feeling sorry for himself or complaining that life isn't fair, David worries most about missing school." I spoke through my tears. "He courageously submits to treatment with a quiet determination. In a different situation I might be filled with motherly pride. Now I have overwhelming pity that I don't want him to see."

"I know," Wayne said. "We'll grieve privately and try to be only an encouragement to David."

"It takes all my control not to cry in front of him. He has to endure enough agony without having to watch mine too."

I'd heard about a six-year-old leukemia patient who made her mother promise not to cry when she visited. The little girl could handle receiving the treatment, but not watching her mom cry. "At least we can spare David that," I said.

"That's right," Wayne answered. "Pity's a destroyer. We can't waste our energy or David's." Wayne took my hand and prayed. "God, please help David get through this. Give us the wisdom we need minute by minute, heal him by whatever means you choose."

At 9 p.m. we picked David up. He couldn't drive for 24 hours after the anesthesia. Easing his tired body into the car, David said, "My instructor had us take a stress test tonight. I'm amazed at how high I tested these past six months new dorm home, change of work/school site, two major high school project deadlines, recent surgery, very recent!" He smiled grimly.

As a psychotherapist I knew stress was a highly suspicious factor in contributing to the immune malfunction that resulted in sickness. Was this the cause?

"Oh God," I prayed. "If only we could know for sure; perhaps others could be protected from this devastation."

The day after biopsy surgery, Wednesday, the oncologist telephoned. Wayne picked up the extension. "The official diagnosis is acute lymphoblastic lymphoma, a rare form of T-cell cancer. There's no cancer in David's nervous system as evidenced in the spinal fluid, but it has already spread to the bone marrow."

"What does that mean?" I asked holding my breath.

"The cancer is at an advanced stage."

The news was far worse than we'd expected.

"'I've consulted with another doctor at the University of Wisconsin Madison Cancer Clinic also," David's oncologist said. "He concurs with the diagnosis and agrees that treatment must start right away, a 2 and a 1/2 year protocol of radiation and chemotherapy, daily the first thirty days, then tapering off to longer intervals weekly and monthly."

My brain was whirling. "Two and a half years!" A thousand agonizing thoughts flashed past me as the doctor

"Doctor this diagnosis is probably correct," Wayne said, "but we've got to be sure with another consultation after all the misdiagnoses David had earlier."

"Okay, but don't delay. I'd like to start treatment on Saturday."

In the meantime back home I rented the funniest movies we could find - Laurel and Hardy and Abbot and Costello. We'd heard about the importance of humor in healing and didn't want to miss one single avenue.

I said aloud, "Lord, we'll do our part as best as our intelligence allows. The rest is up to you, okay?"

A dear friend offered to help with household errands for us. Another friend drove to Madison and back, a three-hour journey to pick up David's medical data and federal express it to Minnesota's Mayo Clinic. Their team of doctors would evaluate David's diagnosis and review the protocol before any treatment began.

This was the beginning of our efforts to seek a combination of the best expert medical knowledge in the field added to the power of God through continual prayer. It was also the start of the work of God's army of saints both sides of heaven to intervene for David's healing.

People began to call immediately with titles of books, names of doctors, the location of information sources. Two dear, retired gentlemen from our community came to explain to David the importance of taking Vitamin C during treatment and for sustaining recovery. They brought David a big jar of it so he could begin taking massive does of Vitamin C immediately. Some of these people we scarcely knew. Many promised to pray and I'm sure they did. David no longer cared who knew as long as they were praying.

We spent the next days collecting data from medical library textbooks. When and why prescribed protocol sometimes didn't work, no one seemed to know for sure. "God, guide us," became my constant prayer.

I learned that people often become an expert in the type of cancer that afflicts them or their loved one.

David's doctor had said, "Cancer treatment is constantly changing state of the art medicine. Before the textbooks can be written, experimental procedures are changed." Even the cancer hotline (I-800-CANCER) of national computerized information can't be kept completely up-to date."

Thursday night, when the hubbub of the day ended, familiar feelings of fear returned. I tried to relinquish them and control my flyaway thoughts.

The anxiety was there when I awakened in the morn. I wanted to pass into oblivion again, and find out life wasn't this crazy nightmare.

Wayne was already up dressing for work. He sat on the bed and took my hand for morning prayer. Each day it was our custom to pray briefly for the children one by one. Now when we came to David, the prayer was intense. I looked at Wayne's strained face.

"It hurts so much doesn't it, Darling," I said emphatically.

Wayne agreed. "At least we're equipping ourselves for battle! We're never going to stop working and praying for David's total healing," he said determinedly.

"Amen." I squeezed his hand tightly. My questions about prayer returned. Could, would prayer work today? Did we have a right to ask? We resolved to make Christian prayer and pastoral contact also part of our search. So much to learn, so little time.

In the meantime and always, we looked for the Lord's joy in each day. Weeks earlier David had auditioned for a part in a TV movie being filmed locally at his place of employment. His big acting debut had arrived. Cancer or not, he had a day off before treatment and in the heavenly realm of coincidence, this happened to be the long-awaited filming day.

CHAPTER 5

At 8 a.m. the next morning we approached Nippersink Resort. On-lookers were milling around in an excited hubbub thirsting for a glimpse of the big stars, Ed Asner and Gary Cole.

When we entered the massive lobby where the chosen cast of extras was congregating, a hush fell among David's fellow summer employees. Obviously, word of his illness had spread. Some acquaintances ignored us. Others approached us with safe, small talk. Perhaps they were waiting for me to bring up the subject. How I wondered would I say, Hi! My son has cancer. What's new with you?

A new awareness hit me that day. There's a physical and social aspect to cancer. Because cancer had happened to David, people couldn't deny it could happen to them. As much as David was liked, his illness made some friends shy away from him.

Cancer divides people who are comfortable with the prospect of their own death from those who aren't. And it identifies those who can deal with difficult personal emotions while they discuss a sensitive subject.

A member of the country club, who had come to watch the filming, ran up to David with a hug saying, "You're so brave." She immediately broke down crying.

David speechlessly extricated himself from her clinging arms.

"I'm so sorry," she said.

He fidgeted and made an excuse to get away.

Oh dear, I thought, she has him dead and wrapped in burial cloths. How discouraging.

I became irritated with people who either saw David as a walking dead man or went to the opposite extreme by trying to pretend that nothing unusual was occurring.

The mother in me broiled with frustration. I couldn't help David! Nobody but God could protect him from the pain of human reactions.

The assistant movie director bounced in and out of the lobby. He'd point silently at extras he wanted for the next scene as if selecting slaves from a market. "That man, the woman in the flowered dress, no not you, the woman next to you. That's it." Then he'd stride off.

His aide was left behind to explain to the privileged, selected few the details of their minuscule parts. Everyone in the lobby had been "promised" a role, but only those actually selected by the regal director's arm would be in the movie.

By 2 p.m. David still hadn't been selected. I began to pray. *Lord, this is really important to Dave. Please get him a chance to act.* Finally about 3:30, the aide ordered all remaining extras to the lakefront cottage for outdoor scenes. The assistant director tapped David's shoulder. "You'll row a background boat that will be visible outside the picture window as we shoot the lead characters arguing inside the cottage."

The aide led David and a middle-aged woman into the roped off filming area. Fortunately, I couldn't see the scene. David had to row 100 yards back and forth four times until the leads got the scene right. Afterwards, he was exhausted, but pleased with his performance. What a ham! For a few hours we could almost but never quite forget what we were up against.

Later that day the Mayo Clinic staff confirmed the diagnosis: acute lymphoblastic lymphoma at an advanced stage and agreed with the suggested protocol.

We scheduled treatment for Saturday. Because the first intravenous chemotherapy treatment can create a shock-like explosion in the body, David had to be hospitalized.

His sister and brother-in-law, Tamara and Greg, who had been checking David's progress by telephone daily from their home in Michigan, arrived on Friday along with our daughter Pam. Two of our very dearest friends, Tom and Pat Cavenagh, also came to visit and support us the night before. Cancer had scared us all. Everyone who loved David wanted to see him and touch him, as if they could help him hold onto life.

After a lovely dinner that Pat brought, we gathered in the living room to enjoy the brilliant glow of the sizzling fire. David sat upon the sofa bed as we clustered around him.

"I think I'll sit here on top of David," Tamara joked.

Pam snuggled up next to him. "You make a great pillow."

Our family had always made little jokes and teased to loosen tension during completely serious moments. Humor is definitely one of God's greatest gifts.

In a serious vein, Wayne suggested, "If prayer is as powerful as Scripture says, and we believe it is, we need to pray now for David's healing." He pulled out the Bible and read Chapter Five from the book of James, verses 14 and 15.

"Is anyone among you sick? He should summon the elders of the church, and they should pray over him and anoint [him] in the name of the Lord, and the prayer of faith will save the sick person, and the Lord will raise him up. If he has committed any sins, he will be forgiven."

We were elders in our church, as were Tom and Pat in theirs. We all laid our hands on different parts of David's body, head, chest, arms, and legs, wherever David had pain, and took turns praying aloud. Wayne started. "Heavenly Father, loving Jesus and powerful Holy Spirit, we ask for Your healing power upon our son David. Lord, we presume to ask, not because of any merit on our part that makes us worthy. But because we remember your promises to us, given when you walked the earth. "Greater power than I have, I will give unto you.'" "Ask anything in my name and it shall be done unto you."

I continued, "Jesus, we have such great love in our hearts for David. We know that love is tiny compared to the love you have for him. We ask that you would lift this terrible illness from his body either miraculously before his chemotherapy treatment starts tomorrow, or else heal him through medical means, but we are united in our request that David have the fullness of health restored to him."

Our friend Tom added, "Lord, we are gathered in your name, and you are present. You said, 'When two or more agree concerning anything on earth, it shall be done.' Lord, we ask in agreement for David's healing."

Our son-in-law, Greg, prayed with a commanding voice. "Satan, source of sickness, we rebuke you from David's body."

Strong words, but yes, I agreed. This cursed cancer had come from the devil himself. I never liked focusing much on Satan, preferring to keep myself turned to Jesus, but I never doubted the devil was real.

I thought about the amazing miraculous signs performed by Jesus, and His incredible promises to His followers, to us, that we, too, should have the power.

One after another we said a spontaneous prayer aloud and acknowledged the presence of God among us. We knew that God doesn't always work miraculously, but sometimes He does.

It was like ... here we are Lord ... remember us? Wayne said, "We're your people, we're depending on your Scripture promises. Every time someone asked you Lord, and believed that you could do it, you healed them. And Lord, we're believing."

Our prayer ended with, "Thank you Jesus for hearing us and for caring! Amen." After hugs and goodnights, we prepared for bed. I experienced a greater peacefulness than I'd known in many days and an expectancy, too. I never doubted for a moment there was a God who heard every word. I know He had the power available to do what we asked. But would He?

CHAPTER 6

Saturday morning dawned bright and clear. Our family breakfast could have seemed normal, if any of us could forget where we were going afterward. Piling into two cars with our overnight gear, the entire family left for St. Mary's Hospital, Madison. We had a real sense of hopefulness hesitant, but looking for a miracle. Why not?

David had never been in a hospital overnight before. Wayne and I decided to stay with him. We'd entered the unknown, frightening, strange world of cancer protocol. It was like visiting a foreign land where we didn't know the language or culture. Deep down we feared we might lose David that first night of treatment. David's two older sisters and younger brother arranged to come also. When we arrived Wayne said to David's oncologist, "Before you begin, we want you to take another x-ray."

"It's not necessary," he said.

Wayne and I realized we sounded foolish to the doctor, but didn't care.

"We want you to x-ray his chest again anyway." I repeated patiently.

"I know what the x-ray will show."

Fully aware that he'd think we were nuts, we said, "David had prayer for healing last night, and we want to know if there's any change in his condition."

To humor us, the doctor finally agreed.

We waited filled with hope. He returned with a tolerant, but kind expression. "No change."

God, where's our miracle? I was disappointed, but tried not to let it show for David's sake. I was genuinely surprised that the mass was still present in David's chest so great had been my faith. I'd been thinking to myself, Lord, this can be a wonderful miraculous healing. I'll tell the whole world what you've done! Well, that wasn't the way God chose to work. Not then, although we believe that He sometimes still does heal like this.

OK, we'd proceed with trusting in God's healing through treatment.

Just then, Tamara's husband, Greg said, "Well the x-ray results don't matter, if you don't see healing yet you still believe. And you show your faith by not receiving treatment."

Wayne and I looked at each other in amazement.

We knew he and Tamara had also been studying the subject of healing. On their eight-hour drive to our home the day before, they'd read aloud a faith-strengthening book, *Christ the Healer* by F. F. Bosworth. This was the basis of their strong comments.

"No way, we need to see medical evidence of healing, otherwise we go through with what God's given us, which is chemotherapy and radiation," I insisted.

Greg quoted Mark 11: 24, "Therefore I tell you, all that whatsoever you ask for in prayer believe that you will receive it and it will be yours." He continued, "Believe first that ye may receive."

We had a lengthy discussion about this in the hall while David's doctor waited to begin the protocol, almost a family argument. This occurred outside an elderly female patient's room and a young AIDS patient's room. The woman passed away later that evening, and the young man soon thereafter. Perhaps this talk about believing and trusting was partly for their benefit.

It certainly wasn't for mine. I couldn't believe what I was hearing! "Greg! Cancer has finally been correctly diagnosed. For four months, we've done nothing that was medically appropriate, and David got worse and worse. Now finally we're about to start treatment and you want us to skip it. God had his chance to heal David without medical intervention. We need to use medicine and prayer now."

Wayne and I were in complete agreement, but David was confused by his brother-in-law Greg's persuasive argument. As a new bride, Tamara was trying to support her husband's opinion. This was too much for me.

I wanted to be tolerant, but Greg was a young Christian and hadn't had experiences like our own in which healing prayers were answered differently than hoped for. We couldn't let there be any block to David's receiving every opportunity medicine and God could offer.

David's sister Pam said, "Greg, you're interfering with my parents. I know you're not a Christian Scientist, but that's how you sound. You haven't the wisdom they have and you need to respect their decision."

Wayne made the final decision. "Greg, we can't agree with you. The doctor is waiting. Let's get under way."

David was willing to accede and begin the treatment.

"God can heal David with treatment or without," Greg said, "but it's right, of course, that David act in obedience to you."

Artistically inclined, Greg spent the rest of the afternoon with Tamara's help making drawings and Bible posters for David's room. These played a part in keeping David's spirits up and were a reminder of faith. One Bible poster proclaimed the verse, "Whatsoever you shall ask in My name, that will I do, that the Father may be glorified in the Son. If you shall ask anything in my name, I will do it. (John 14:13,14)

Greg also drew a picture of David giving a speech in the year 2010 with Jesus at His side explaining to a large audience how God had healed him of cancer 25 years ago. The inscription at the bottom was Proverbs 3:13,16: "Happy (blessed) is the man that finds wisdom. Long life is in her right hand, and in her left hand riches and honor.'"

Tamara and Greg, Pam and Dan all slept in a hospital guest room on the floor below. Wayne and I slept together on one twin cot in David's room, the only size bed that could fit into the small space.

I lay awake most of the night trying to keep from falling off the bed and waiting for the "explosion" in David's body which didn't occur, thank God! David tolerated his first chemotherapy well. After Saturday and Sunday treatment and observation, we all headed home.

The counterattack had begun!

More chemotherapy followed in the next days and weeks and some of it was injected directly into David's spinal column. This procedure caused David incredible pain and excruciating headaches. Afterwards I brought him to the hospital emergency room. David lost any typical eighteen-year-old self-consciousness. He writhed on the floor while waiting to be checked. David's oncologist prescribed morphine. However, even this didn't control the pain.

Before the next injection two weeks later, David's doctor announced, "We'll try changing administration procedures. Instead of performing the spinal tap as an outpatient in my office, David will be hospitalized so that following the procedure he can lie perfectly still for eight hours until his spinal fluid stabilizes."

"After eight hours in the hospital, I drove David home in our van with him lying flat on a makeshift bed in the back.

The next day, as he tried to get up, David cried out, "Mom, I can't handle this. The pain is back! I thought I'd already had the worst pain a person could feel, but this is worse than anything I've had!"

The horrible pain lasted about ten days, just until David was due for another spinal chemotherapy treatment. Next the doctor tried changing the type of chemical he was injecting. That didn't work either. The doctor was obviously puzzled. It was as though David was paralyzed a week at a time because he couldn't move without tremendous pain. Nothing had helped. Pain itself was not a foreign experience to David. He said, "If it's just getting through the pain, I can probably do it. Not knowing what the chemical is doing to my brain and spinal column when this unexplainable reaction occurs scares me. The doctor said that spinal chemotherapy treatment is not normally painful."

David's faith in doctors visibly diminished further.

The oncologist consulted with his associates to try to come up with a solution and called us back. "Mr. and Mrs. Rolfs, the neurosurgeon's suggestion, and the one I recommend, is to perform brain surgery to put a shunt directly into David's brain for the infusion of the required chemotherapy into his spinal column. Inserting the chemical directly may alleviate the pain."

"May?" Wayne and I asked in unison.

In the next breath, the oncologist said, "There's no guarantee that this will solve the problem." One of those malpractice insurance precautionary statements for self-protection? This verifies doctors are not responsible for producing outcomes - comments like this made too frequently strip away patient confidence.

When David heard this recommendation, he was angry.

The doctor had stated honestly that the brain surgery was still not as perfected as he'd like. There were definite dangers. Still, the doctor encouraged David to continue with the two-and-one-half year treatment procedure with intermittent spinal chemotherapy treatments.

David said, "I see myself as a potential vegetable healed of cancer, but going into in a coma and dying."

He was confused and angry. "Nobody has any answers. I'm a guinea pig!" he vented.

By this time David already had five weeks of treatment behind him. We were in the midst of a fall season that was never more beautiful. As the golden glow came over the huge oak and hickory trees, David struggled over his decision whether to continue with the spinal chemotherapy.

He had to sign a surgical permission statement himself because he was eighteen. Technically he was in remission; what a sweet word that became. The lumps on his head were gone, as was the tumor in his chest. A recent bone marrow biopsy showed no sign of any cancer cells.

After weighing the brain surgery option David said, "Now a dangerous surgical procedure is being recommended without any assurance it will work. The operation itself might kill me. Mom and Dad, I'm considering discontinuing the spinal treatments. My doctor can't explain what's causing this complication. Why don't doctors know?" He groaned helplessly. "Look what their bumbling around had already cost me. If I'd been correctly diagnosed sooner, the cancer might have been stopped before it entered my bone marrow."

We couldn't deny the truth of what he said. We put in a call to his doctor and over the phone asked if David could continue with only the non-spinal aspects of chemotherapy treatment: oral prednisone and IV injections of powerful chemotherapy drugs listed in his protocol, vincristine and Adriamycin."

The oncologist answered abruptly. "There's no point. It's an all or nothing procedure that needs to be followed precisely. Spinal injections are essential. I can't treat him any other way."

That evening after dinner, we gave David the latest information. "The protocol must be followed exactly as it's been designed for two and a half years."

David was terribly discouraged.

"Son, the final decision is yours. We can only counsel you."

"How soon does he need to know?" David asked.

"Before the next scheduled spinal in five days."

CHAPTER 7

The scene seemed strangely out-of-kilter; something distant and elusive tickled my memory. It was a still, crisp October evening. We sat cozily around the steady orange-gold display of our wood-burning fireplace, Wayne and I on the comfy, pillow-backed sofa, David in the Lazy-boy reading, and Dan stretched out on the floor doing homework.

The three pumpkins David bought that day were lined up like sentinels waiting to be carved. Indian corn and a burlap and straw scarecrow decorated the front door. The delicious fragrance of popcorn floated through the house.

Suddenly I knew what seemed weird. This night resembled old times, pleasant family nights before our carefree attitude had been attacked by the specter of cancer among us.

Wayne grimaced as pictures of one world tragedy after another paraded across the TV screen.

I said, "We've come a long way from the perfection of the Garden of Eden, haven't we. Destructive pollution, greed and illness permeate our world. And now we're feeling the ravage of disease firsthand." I looked over at David.

How much like an old man he appeared with his nearly baldhead bent over a book. Day by day, his hair fell I out in clumps as he slept. The first morning it happened he called me in and pointed silently at the soft brown strands he found on his pillow when he awoke.

I'd said, "How about saving your hair in an envelope for a ceremonial burning and then tossing the ashes to the wind? What's too painful to mourn, we'll celebrate somehow." The Lord only knows where I got that idea.

David said, "Mom, that's ridiculous."

About a week later, I saw David alone in the yard one evening burning clumps of his hair on the ground.

Typically eighteen, he said, "I want to be normal, Mom, like other guys." He despised the new wig-crown of difference he wore in public. It seemed unnatural and uncomfortable despite the protests of friends like Scott who said, "David, we can hardly tell you're wearing a hairpiece."

David's head shone tonight in the soft lamplight. I turned my attention to the laundry that needed folding. Perhaps sensing that I'd been studying him, David looked up with a brightness in his eyes. "Mom, Dad, I'm reading *Christ the Healer* by F. F. Bosworth." His voice hesitated.

"That's the book Tamara and Greg brought you, isn't it?"

"Yes, Bosworth describes God's healing role as revealed in Scripture. The concept makes a lot of sense to me although I've never heard it before."

"What do you mean?" Wayne asked, clearly intrigued. We'd been churchgoers for years, and David had never balked at attending, too. What principle might David have discovered that he hadn't been previously taught?

"Dad, it's pretty straightforward for me. But I'd like to know what you and Mom think. Jesus died for me, right?"

"Yes," we answered in unison. David had heard that hundreds of times.

"By His death on the cross Jesus broke the power of sin and sickness. Sickness entered the world simultaneously with sin. Jesus atoned for both."

David went on to explain that during His life on earth, Jesus healed everyone who called on Him and believed He could heal and forgive sin. David's words tumbled out with more enthusiasm than I'd seen since before his diagnosis. "Do you see what that means? God loves me and wants me healed!"

When David stopped for breath, Wayne said, "Son, we all love you and want you well! I don't have to read a book to know that."

"But, Dad, I believe it's also God's desire to heal everyone including me, just as it's His desire that everyone choose to follow Him to heaven. We are freely presented with the gift of salvation to accept or reject by our desire and willingness to believe."

We looked at David with a mixture of love and pity for his naiveté. More than anything we knew David wanted to be free of this cursed disease and we wanted him whole. But was David becoming irrational in his desperate longing for health?

Wayne said, "What about the exceptions, those who aren't healed?" He turned off the TV to give David full attention.

"Because some people aren't saved doesn't mean it isn't God's will for them," David explained carefully. "Just because some people aren't healed doesn't mean it's not God's desire to heal them." David nodded his head for emphasis. "Salvation requires a commitment to trust God. So does healing. God not only wants me healed, He will heal me, if I believe."

If David wasn't our straight "A" son who could reason logically, I would have said he sounded like a fanatic. Wayne and David often had heavy theological or political discussions, but never had the topic been this crucial.

"Wait a minute here," Wayne answered, "you're making healing a condition of faith. How can you measure faith? I can't believe God would refuse to heal someone because they didn't have the right amount of faith."

"Why shouldn't faith be a condition? Salvation depends on faith, not on any measurable quantity, but a willingness to believe. That's enough!" David retorted.

Their voices weren't argumentative, but the tone became more intense. We wanted truth, and if that truth brought the gift of hope, great. If not, none of us wanted to be deceived by a wishful thought, however enticing.

Wayne groped for a logical reply. Finally he said, "I believe God's ways are more complex than that. We're to ask, and if it's part of His plan for our lives, Jesus heals."

My eyes bounced from Wayne to David.

David countered thoughtfully, "We can't understand why some people are never healed. It's not their fault. Nevertheless Jesus is capable of communicating clearly and directs us to pray believing we will receive healing. He hasn't disguised what He expects from us, because He wants us to know His principles for our lives. Many churches today disregard the words of Jesus, 'Amen, amen, I say to you, whoever believes in Me will do the works that I do and will do greater ones than these, because I am going to the Father." (John 14:12, NASB)

We listened amazed at how much thought David had given this.

"Dad, God's people are being robbed by their ignorance. God is sovereign: healing isn't hocus-pocus, hit or miss. What greater works are being done today?" David demanded.

The longer David spoke, the more he convinced himself. "If we're sick, we should live eagerly, prayerfully anticipating our healing. We can't know it's not God's intention to heal us, unless we're dead. No matter how sick, our healing may be just around the corner."

"How I wish it were always true just as you say, but it isn't," I interjected. "I can't explain why, but I've prayed for people who weren't healed, as well as for people who have been."

David flayed his arms like flags in the wind. "That's because people put their faith in medicine alone. We should also use all the logical, natural means God has made available through doctors in addition to exercising supernatural faith. That's the opposite of the passive process of waiting for life or death."

I shook my head thoroughly confused. "This is heavy stuff and it's getting late."

"Mom, Dad, can we talk a little longer?" David said more calmly. "It's important for me to be able to argue this out to be sure my thinking is right. I want to hear your objections, I really do."

David changed tactics and took the offensive. "Why should we bother to ask for healing in our prayers if God is going to work according to His unchangeable plan anyway?" David recounted the Old Testament story of Hezekiah. God sent a messenger to tell him he'd die. Then Hezekiah asked God to heal him. God actually changed his mind and extended the years of Hezekiah's life by fifteen years (Isaiah 38: 1-22, NASB)."

"I'm sure God had His reasons," Wayne countered. "Dad, that's just it, He had good reason," David pointed out. "God was moved by Hezekiah's prayer and belief to change his mind. Mark 11: 24 (NASB) says, 'All things for which you pray and ask, believe that you have received them, and they shall be granted you.' Believe that you may receive,'" David repeated.

"Here we are back to that again. How can you be sure you're believing strongly enough?" Wayne asked.

"I choose the attitude of faith; that's good enough." David jumped up and started pacing the floor. "I'm sure it helps to have a community of believers faithfully praying for you, too, like the friends of the paralyzed man who brought him to Jesus. Sometimes when you're sick, it's hard to pray regularly and faithfully for yourself. I'm grateful for your prayers and those of others who will believe with me."

A moment of silence followed in which I tried to collect my thoughts. I had lots of questions.

"David, what about so called 'faith-healers?' Where do they fit in all this?"

David answered quickly, "If they put the power for healing into the hands of men instead of God, they're wrong."

"I agree with that."

Like the message of Jesus Himself, the ideas David shared were simple, yet highly controversial. Taking a deep breath, David repeated, "Jesus has healing powers and He will intervene in our lives if we ask. Our healing doesn't depend on our good works. None of us are worthy of healing any more than we deserve salvation."

Wayne interjected gently. "God allows sickness in the world, just as He allows sin, for His ultimate glory. 'How unsearchable are His judgments and unfathomable His ways. (Romans 12: 33b)'"

"Right Dad. There's much we don't know, but the consistent healing activity of Jesus without exception makes me think healing someone must bring more glory to God than the continued suffering of His servants. Otherwise why did Jesus heal everyone that asked him?"

David continued. "Why aren't their records of Him saying. 'No. It brings more glory to the Father if you remain sick.' Also why didn't Jesus ever ask the Father first if it was His Father's will to heal a particular person before He performed each healing?" David answered the question himself. "Because He knew healing was the Father's will."

Wayne and I were momentarily speechless. We'd never thought about that.

"Jesus delayed healing Lazarus briefly," David added, "just as He doesn't always heal us immediately, but He never flat out refused to heal. Jesus couldn't perform many healings however when there was a lack of faith, like in his hometown of Nazareth. Mom, Dad, that's what's written. Jesus came to lead us into truth."

"You're saying David," I clarified, "the confidence we have in salvation is the same confidence we should have in believing that we are going to be healed when we ask?"

Patiently David went on as though he were the parent educating us. "Jesus took our sins and sickness away according to Isaiah 53:4,5 and Matthew 8: 16,17. We don't need to understand how salvation works before we ask for it and are forgiven. We believe first and then we experience the effect, the same is true of healing."

My head spun crazily. David ignored some point in his logic, but what? Then I knew. "What about Paul's thorn in the flesh?" I asked.

I might have known he'd already thought that through. David paused to control the strong emotions that were being evoked. Then he explained that the Old Testament reference to thorn in the flesh might not refer to physical sickness, but a messenger of Satan sent to constantly buffet Paul through hardships like shipwreck. Paul's life showed no proof that he made a physical reference. Certainly he lived as a virile, active man. Moses specifically used the same term "thorn in the flesh" to describe the Jews during the Exodus because they complained continually and were a great trial to Moses.

"David, I'll grant that's possible; but we've all got to die some day of something."

He agreed, "But it shouldn't happen before Scripture's stated time in Psalms. The righteous shall live three score and ten years,' maybe longer. With long life I will satisfy him." (Psalm 91).

"David, you know every Christian doesn't live that long," Wayne said.

"Still it's God's best plan. People can use their free will to cut their lives short by an unhealthy lifestyle or by sinful choices that hurt themselves or others, like armed robbery, shooting drugs. We need to live wisely, as God spelled out in the Bible, to protect others and ourselves remaining fully armed and totally prepared." David finished enthusiastically.

David's words sounded scary; I looked at him painfully. Dan had long since gone to bed. We had gotten to the bottom line. Trusting God for his healing wasn't just David's last-ditch, vague maneuver, but his carefully reasoned, viable choice.

Wound up, David didn't stop. "Even medicine is verifying God's Word now, like the fact that laughter and happy thoughts are conducive to healing."

"Right," I said, "Science calls that psychoneuroimmunology."

"Eons ago the Bible said in Proverbs, 'A merry heart-doeth good like medicine,'" David insisted.

I asked one last question. "If all this is true, why aren't more people healed?"

David quoted Hosea. "My people perish for want of knowledge (Hosea 4:6, NASB)."

We wanted David to have the best opportunity for long-term recovery. I couldn't come up with any Scriptural basis for disagreement. A phrase kept running through my mind, "Say but the Word, and I shall be healed. "

Wayne was deep in thought as David finished. "I seem to have run out of medical hope, but I'm sure God can heal me. Before this recent complication, I only had a 50-50 chance anyway with treatment; now I'm trusting God 100%. I'd like to discontinue my protocol with your approval."

So that was it. Wow, was all I could think.
Wayne said, "We need to think and pray on it."
David agreed. "I will too."

CHAPTER 8

The search for wisdom took us deep into the heart of God's Word. How did Jesus perform His miracles? I tried to compose a letter to David explaining what I believed about supernatural healing. I discovered my thoughts weren't as clear as I'd expected.

On one side, David believed strongly in God's healing today. On the other hand we knew David had lost faith in medicine. In truth I had too. If not rose-colored, my thinking was certainly amber-colored. I actually had believed that Disney's Epcot slogans were true: "There's no limit to what man can achieve." "Life is under our control." God relegated earthly power to capable humans. "If an important discovery hadn't yet been made, the incredible mind and ferocious will of humanity's 'brilliants' simply hadn't tried hard enough yet." I had to admit now that this fairy tale of human pride seemed attractive, but false.

Medicine had no miracle to offer. Did God?

Several friends from Illinois recommended a medical doctor who specialized in dietary treatment for cancer. David was interested; perhaps this was part of God's method.

On a blustery fall day we ventured into Evanston, Illinois for an unusual experience. We waited over three hours past our scheduled appointment time. The waiting room reeked of garlic. Some patients had come prepared for their long wait with salads in Tupperware bowls.

When the doctor finally materialized we were led into the examining room; we saw him for five minutes. He was about five-foot-eleven with dark hair, olive skin, and he exuded vitality. With the zeal of a salesman he elaborated, "Diet is the key to health," as he checked the color of David's skin and studied David's hands and feet.

The doctor launched into a non-stop dialogue in a persuasive philosophical tone. "I recommend a macrobiotic diet. Eat foods in their whole, natural state. The general population is unaware of the chemical dangers of eating poultry and daily products. We suggest eating only a couple pieces of bread and fish per week, and absolutely no sugar. The delicate chemical balance within the body must be maintained. The addition of foreign chemicals in food alters their harmonious natural chemical composition. Three times a day practice relaxation and do regular physical exercise. Both are essential to healing."

Eyes glowing with fervor, the doctor quoted various sources and gave us a recent newspaper article endorsing his nutritional philosophy. We were plied with other reading material to help us understand the acid/alkaline balance in foods.

After warm handshakes and a pat on David's back, the doctor bounced off to inspire another patient.

A six-foot tall, skinny medical assistant, who looked like a stalk of celery with a grin on top, came in and drew a huge tube of blood from David. Then he explained the specific dietary procedures the doctor recommended for David's illness including eating various types of seaweed: nori, kombu, arame, and their preparation methods. As the words rolled off the young man's tongue, I craved a butter pecan ice cream cone.

When the medical assistant left David said bitterly, "Goodbye McDonald's and fast food restaurants with my friends." Wayne and I silently noted our son's new loss, familiar and favorite foods.

I never would have thought David would agree to this way of eating, but he did. Some spark of confidence radiated from the nutritional doctor that the oncologist lacked. A desperate, young man doesn't need much hope to stir a responsive chord, but he needs some. Although David put his trust in God for healing, he had no objection to co-operating with any reasonable medical treatment.

In all fairness, this medical doctor never encouraged us to stop chemotherapy, although his written material contained amazing accounts of patients who had been cured with only diet, exercise and relaxation. Clearly diet was a significant factor in health. The doctor's theory held part of the truth, but not all of it.

On the ride home, Wayne said, "David, if you're going to eat these foods, we'll make them our diet too." Dan and I agreed, "Our health will benefit, too, if the doctor's research has merit. But, we'll avoid any Eastern mystical overtones associated with the diet, and focus only on the low fat, high carbohydrate principles." (Months later the American Cancer Society revealed its first research on a similar anticancer diet promoting fresh vegetables and grains.)

At the moment we had no idea what we were getting into. A friend of mine came and taught me to cook macrobiotlcally. Another friend of a friend, herself a cancer patient on the same diet, graciously came and shared her cooking tips.

Our primary drink became kukicha tea, a bark from Japan steeped to release its rich deposit of calcium. All dairy products were out. Making dinner became a two-and-a-half-hour process.

I cooked new foods like soba and udon noodles. We ate vegetable soups with miso, stir-fries and main dishes like cauliflower spaghetti. Our sandwich spread, a pureed lentil bean dish, was crushed and flavored with lemon and tamari. Our flavorings were garlic, sea salt, and tamari. Dan often excused himself before our limited dessert repertoire of sugar-free apple, pumpkin or squash pie.

David also continued the regime of extensive vitamins he'd already begun.

Perhaps the main benefit of the macrobiotic diet was our laughter at dinner every night over the food's strange appearance and texture. One night Wayne said, "This isn't too bad, tonight."

I quickly said, "You're right. It's tasty in its own way."

David mocked our enthusiasm. "Yeah, this is great. Have a little more bark tea with your seaweed soup, Dad."

And Dan added, "Can we have seconds on the barley 'meat' loaf, mom, huh, mom, please?"

If God, food and exercise could keep David in remission we'd know.

Too soon the time came for another injection of chemotherapy into David's spine. We still hadn't come to the conclusion that David should discontinue medical treatment. Perhaps to placate us David struggled through the procedure.

He had a third painful, frightening aftermath. Afterwards, David announced firmly, 'I'm trusting in God and natural means to keep me well. I have no other reasonable option."

I can't say we were in 100% agreement, but we had nothing better to offer. Knowing David was presently in remission, however temporary, helped. We understood his concerns and promised to support him all the way. The oncologist tried to talk David out of his decision to discontinue chemotherapy. David, like his Dad, appeared easy-going, but once David firmly made up his mind, he was unmovable.

We studied Scripture to learn the meaning of "standing in the gap," giving David the strength of our own belief especially during those moments of human weakness, when his faith might grow thin. It meant faithful prayers and trust in a healing God.

David's strong conviction had been born of young faith and medical desperation. Believing and trusting became extremely difficult at times. Our cultural environment doesn't often recognize the supernatural power of God or the simplicity of diet and exercise as healing tools.

Peter, the husband of a friend and a non-denominational minister, offered to help. "Tell David I'm standing in faith with him for God's healing. I look forward to meeting him."

In the months ahead, Peter became a frequent visitor who taught David much about God. Above all he stressed how important it was for David to desire a deeper relationship with Jesus Christ more than anything else, even more than healing.

David needed this strong adult support. When doing errands in our little town, often somebody would approach David and say, "Has the cancer come back yet?"

Through fall into winter, David continued to enjoy school, a trite phrase, but 100% true. He'd moved home and become a commuter-student at the University of Wisconsin-Whitewater less than an hour away. We resisted the temptation to think bitterly of other young people who found school boring and cut classes frequently. Many a day during his previous chemo all David could manage was to get to school for a couple hours, return, and collapse. Some days he couldn't make it at all. I went instead and took notes for him. November and December passed with David desperately trying to catch up. He'd dropped two courses, but was salvaging three.

One day when he returned home from school David read a registered letter from his oncologist saying, "You'll be dead within a year without further treatment." He claimed David's cancer was extremely aggressive and wasn't eliminated from the little treatment he'd already had.

David reacted angrily. "I can't believe a doctor would send me this lousy letter. His medical treatment had poor prognosis and unexplainable complications. The doctor wrote this when he had no decent alternative to offer." David's determination against cancer treatment and his disillusionment with doctors intensified.

Occasionally David visited his former teachers at high school. David explained his reliance on God's healing to them. I'd hear David on the phone telling friends the medical route wasn't working. Then he'd describe his belief in God's healing power. To humor David or possibly out of astonishment, no one openly disagreed or tried to dissuade him. Yet their eyes often displayed pity and a lack of belief.

Christmas, always a special family time, was wonderful in 1985. We were all alive and together. Christ was real; no other gifts were needed in our lives. Christmas morning, as usual, Wayne, the children and I visited the patients at the county nursing home. David read "The Night Before Christmas" with vivid dramatic effects for a group of elderly ladies who had gathered around him. I watched with parental pride and a silent prayer that we'd be there together again the following year.

At the very end of December, David called me into the bathroom. "What's this do you suppose?" He showed me a swollen lump on his head.

"David, I don't know what the lump is, but we'll pray for it to go away. Would you like to see a doctor and get it checked?"

"No!" David answered emphatically. "Perhaps Satan is tempting me to unbelief with this sign. After all Satan can perform signs and wonders, too."

I wasn't surprised at David's reaction. He had no confidence left in internists or oncologists. He chose the walk of faith. Yet deep down I sensed he was a little scared.

I wasn't comfortable with not having it examined. Yet it was too soon to say if this one tiny lump was a symptom of the return of cancer, or just a bump, an infected hair follicle. One week later something happened that took our minds totally off the ominous bump.

CHAPTER 9

Thursday, January 7th David's friends, Mark and Scott, dropped in to watch 'IV. They left after the 10 p.m. news, and David grabbed his insulated jacket. "I won't be gone long, mom; it's too cold," David called over his shoulder as he hurried out.

His health regimen called for frequent exercise and David particularly liked to jog in the stillness of late evening with God and the stars as company. Afterwards he sometimes spent time alone at the lakefront.

I snuggled into bed to read, and fell asleep instantly.

About thirty minutes later there was a loud knock on the front door. Wayne opened to a Delavan Township policeman who announced hurriedly, "Your son's been hit by a car driven by a drunk driver."

"What?" Wayne gasped.

The officer went on. "The report came in by radio. David's alive, but he's been hurt, how badly I don't know. The man who hit him brought him to Lakeland Hospital. I'll meet you in the emergency room."

Wayne said, "We'll be right there!"

He came into our bedroom and awakened me. "David's hurt."

"Hurt," I said, coming out of a sleepy fog. "Of course, he has cancer."

"No, he's been hit by a car!"

"This is a terrible joke," I began. From Wayne's white, shocked face I knew it wasn't. My next thought was David's dead. "Oh no!" I moaned.

Wayne reassured me, "There's been an accident, but he's alive."

I jumped up and started shaking so badly I dropped back on the bed. "I can't believe it," I said dumbly.

"I'm going to the hospital. You'd better stay with Daniel in case he wakes up."

"No. I'll call someone to stay with him. I'm coming. I just have to sit a minute before I can move." Wayne wrapped his arms around me and held me tight. We were both shaking by then.

He released me quickly. "While you throw on some clothes, I'll call Peter for prayer support."

Our minister friend expressed shock, and then said, "I'll meet you at the hospital."

I called my dear widowed friend Ruth to stay with thirteen-year-old Daniel in case he woke up.

"Stay as long as necessary," she said. "I'll spend the night; I'll be right over, just leave the door open."

During the fifteen-minute ride to the hospital, I kept asking God, How could you let this happen? We're praying for a healing, and now this? Aren't we getting through to you?

Two Scripture verses I'd read or heard somewhere came to me. "What man has meant for evil, God will turn to good." (Genesis 50:20) and "All things work together for good for those who love the Lord." (Romans 8:28). I didn't understand how this accident, on top of what David had already experienced, could ever be used for good.

But deep down, in the God-place of my heart, I knew that I would trust Him again. Trust was easy when every-thing went my way. It became a commitment of the will, when life seemed to be falling apart.

Walking into the emergency room, we braced ourselves for whatever we might find. We still struggled with disbelief wanting to awaken from this new nightmare. Policemen milled about as we walked back into the treatment area looking for David. A staff person hurried over to direct us.

From a distance we saw David propped on a sheet-covered cot. His eyes darted about anxiously to see what was going to happen next. Emergency room nurses and doctors flustered about him. David's face lit up feebly when he saw us.

"Hi," David said in a whispery voice of pain. I hugged him gently trying to avert my eyes from the red splotches that seemed to be everywhere.

The left pant leg of his spattered jeans had been cut with a scissors exposing a bloody mass of flesh. I couldn't look at it directly yet. David's two formerly white, blood-spotted tennis shoes had been set neatly at the foot of the cot. These were the only order in the seeming chaos.

I blinked rapidly at the sight of David lying in the midst of new pain and turmoil. Squeezing his hand, I said with my jaw set firmly, "You're going to be alright."

The words of assurance again! "Faith is the assurance of things hoped for." (Hebrews 11: 1, Amp.) I spoke sincerely, "On the way here God has impressed upon me the verse, 'What man has done as evil, God will use for good,' just as in the story of Joseph in the Book of Genesis."

David was fully conscious. Although dazed he understood me. That verse of confirmation, that God had not abandoned him, no matter how terrible the circumstances, seemed to calm him.

The nurse asked, "Are you David's parents?" Then she explained, "David Is being prepared for immediate surgery. His leg x-rays show multiple breaks. He has a concussion and scattered cuts and bruises."

A policeman introduced himself and explained, "Apparently the car swerved off the road and hit David with the front right fender throwing him through the air some distance. The man that hit him is in the waiting room. He already apologized to David, but wants to see him again."

The nurse went on, "The driver claimed he tried to get help from a home nearby, but no one answered his knock. He went back to where he hit David, dragged him into the back seat of his car, and drove him here."

She paused for breath, and added as an aside to us, "Thank God your son didn't have a broken back. Moving him could have been fatal. Instead of stopping at the police station two blocks away, the driver brought David all the way here." The nurse shook her head in amazement.

"I didn't know what was happening," David told us. "I wondered if I was being kidnapped. The man said he was taking me to a hospital, but I didn't know if I could believe him. He drove wildly swerving all over the roads. I was worried I'd be killed in the car. At the hospital he told me to get out, and I hopped in on one leg as fast as I could."

"David's broken bone was protruding through his skin," added the sympathetic ER nurse. "It's a wonder he didn't go into shock. The orthopedic surgeon is on his way. Your MD is already here and scrubbing up to assist."

"Thank you," we managed to mumble.

Pastor Peter arrived minutes later. His short, muscular frame and deep voice filled with concern encouraged us. He brought a heightened air of God's peace into David's curtained-off cubicle.

An indifferent young, policeman with a cold, impersonal attitude, took a statement from David bit by bit. We learned the drunk driver had been returning home from bowling. Next the policeman brought in the burly driver with his half-buttoned shirt hanging out of his pants. A smell of stale smoke and liquor mingled with the hospital antiseptic making me nauseous.

60

Suddenly sober and crying, the man grabbed David's hand and wouldn't let go. He repeated over and over, "I'm sorry."

David said, "That's alright. I'm glad you didn't leave me there in the cold."

Hospital staff and police seemed to be waiting for some kind of scene. No way, I thought, "Go your way, your sins are forgiven, seemed too easy," but Jesus said it. I sighed knowing we'd deal with the consequences of this man's actions a long time. I numbly swept away my anger. What good would bitterness do? Wayne and I knew that forgiveness doesn't mean the aftermath of pain disappears, only that it becomes manageable in the comfort of Christ.

We sincerely told the driver, "We're grateful you didn't leave David at the accident site where he might have frozen or bled to death."

The policeman asked more questions. We couldn't care less about these issues now. Later we heard this same driver had a previous record of drunk driving, and had been let off without penalty, which disturbed us. We've never seen him since, but we have prayed for him many times. Supposedly he carried only minimal insurance, had a handicapped child, and modest resources. We chose not to sue even though a large financial settlement might have been some comfort to David for all his pain.

Before David went into the operating room, the surgeon explained David's condition in detail. "Your son's leg has been broken in numerous places, shattered is probably a more accurate word. He has other cuts and bruises that will heal with time. The leg is our most pressing concern. During this first operation we'll clean the site to prevent infection, and prepare to reset the bones. We think we can save the leg, but it's questionable if he'll ever walk without a limp."

Our spirits slumped. *Oh Lord, this too?*

Peter offered to stay with us during the two-hour surgery and helped us lift our hearts to the Lord. We wept off and on and questioned God. We told Peter sadly, "David has a tiny swelling on his head that he's choosing to ignore. It mayor may not be the return of cancer. David refuses to consult his oncologist in light of his past inability to deal satisfactorily with his complications. Anyway, at this point David is relying totally on God and good health habits for his continued remission."

"I see," Peter said. "And you?"

"We're not comfortable with David's refusal to maintain medical contact. He harbors strong anger toward his oncologist for sending him a registered letter that he'll be dead by the end of the year if he doesn't have more chemotherapy," Wayne said.

I interjected. "David's eighteen and legally must sign for treatment. We trust God, but we want to see the reality of His healing power. We don't need to deny our senses and pretend David's fine if he isn't. "

Peter listened carefully before replying, "David has committed his life to Christ. We have God's word that He will heal those who are His. We must keep our minds and hearts on Christ, and not on what we see. Remember faith is the assurance of things 'unseen.'"

I smiled faintly. "I already used that verse tonight."

Wayne pulled a folded piece of worn notebook paper from his wallet. "I think I understand. Every day I read these thoughts I've written. I believe this is what God is saying through his word."

Wayne read, "Do not just believe in my power, love, healing, peace. Accept it, receive it. It's for you, my son, now. Don't block it by your doubts, fears, and worries. Let it flow into you and into David, fill you and heal."

I listened scarcely breathing, wanting so badly for this to happen to our son.

Wayne went on, "All things are possible through Me. If you focus on illness and difficulties you will receive them—if you focus on Me and on My Word you will not block my healing powers, my strength, peace, and joy. Surrender fully to faith in me and what I can do for you. You cannot do this, but I can. You are healed.'"

"Are?" I questioned.

Wayne wrote his response to God beneath. "Thank you for your mercy, love, compassion. Jesus, I love you. I receive in loving thanks your healings and gifts."

I understood. Not doubting was a commitment of the will, but I wasn't sure I could do it.

Shortly after 4:00 a.m. the surgery was over. David remained asleep from the anesthetic. We drove home and flopped into bed totally exhausted.

The next day we called our other children with the news. They were shocked. Pam said, "Mom, Dad, what's happening to our family? It's as if there's a satanic attack going on. What next?"

"I don't know Pam," I answered "but we refuse to stop trusting God just because we're going through tragedies. He's brought us through the good times. We're going to trust Him in these tough times."

We again checked the possessions in our house, in David's bedroom, his war games and books, to remove anything that might offend the Lord. We even anointed our computer with a dab of oil. We prayed for the Lord to bring us through this latest tragedy.

In the days following surgery David was in considerable pain. His back and neck injuries from the accident were almost as excruciating as the leg pain. Other than anesthetic during surgery, David refused all pain medication. He feared that the chemical substances would upset the delicate balance of his immune system and cause the cancer to return.

I cooked all of David's macrobiotic meals at home, and transported them to the hospital so David could stay on his chemical-free diet.

Visits of many relatives and friends helped make these two weeks of hospitalization bearable. Wayne, Dan, David's brother, and I visited David dally. Dan began to view hospital sunrooms as his alter living rooms. He learned to do his homework with the blare of a loudspeaker system in the background, never once complaining.

When David felt up to it he and Dan played board games. David's sister, Pam, spent several nights sleeping on the floor next to his hospital bed. Our family fought for David with our love, our presence and our prayers.

During the second operation on his leg, we prayed the bones could be set without placing a permanent rod in David's leg. The Lord answered that prayer. David wore a beret given him by our Catholic priest friend, Father Vojtek, to cover the small lump still on his head. David was trusting God alone to heal him of cancer and refused to be examined by an oncologist.

CHAPTER 10

Weeks before David's accident, when he appeared to be stable, Wayne and I planned to attend the national Professional Golfer's Association Show in Orlando, Florida for two days. Immediately following that, we'd also accepted the invitation of friends for a six-day vacation retreat at their condo in the Cayman Islands. I happened to mention to my wonderful Christian friend, Jeanette, that we were canceling our plans because of David's accident.

Jeanette said gently, "You and Wayne need this time.

"Wayne looks like he's ready to drop," she said gently. I probably did too, but she kindly didn't say that to my face. "You go," she insisted. "I'll come over each day to give David his meals and vitamins and bathe him. Perhaps you can get family members to spend the night with him, and I'll handle the days. Don't worry about a thing!"

I had mixed feelings about leaving. I wanted to stay with David, but I knew we could both use a rest. Our college age daughter, Pam, and both sets of our parents offered to take turns spending nights with David.

"That settles it," Wayne said. "We're going if David is released from the hospital on schedule." He made arrangements to get our passports.

We had another reason for wanting to go. David's best friend through grade school, Ricky, moved to Orlando four years ago. To our horror we received word that seventeen-year-old Ricky had developed cancer of the lymph system, Hodgkin's disease, a few months after David's diagnosis. We wanted to visit Ricky and his parents.

I wondered if the cancer of our boys who'd been separated for years had an environmental cause. If so, what? We ruled out golf courses even though both fathers were in the golf profession, because David and Ricky were almost never at the golf course. They spent many hours playing at our local lake, which was often treated with chemicals for water clarity. Was this the cause? The latency effect of various chemicals can be up to ten years before the immune system weakens and signs of cancer appear.

We shuddered to think of our children as mysterious victims of unidentified carcinogens. We'll probably never know the exact cause.

The day of David's hospital release arrived. Another pastor friend, David Hawley, came and anointed David with oil for healing before he went home. I prepared lists of instructions to be followed during our absence, while Wayne picked David up from the hospital.

I watched David hobble through the door in a toe-to-hip cast and collapse on the living room sofa bed.

In David's weakened condition, leaning on his crutches was a strain. Even a trip to the bathroom was a major effort.

My son. My son ... I prayed silently and an answer came into my thoughts. *"His ordeal isn't as bad as My Son's on the cross."*

We made David as comfortable as possible, pushing the furniture against the walls to make wide pathways for his crutches, and placing books and 'IV within easy reach.

David's sister, Pam, arrived to take the first shift of his care. Like a fairy princess she always carried joy with her gentle smile and energy that transfused everyone around her.

"Pam, you're exactly the person David needs," I said.

Overhearing us in the next room, David said irritably. "Mom and Dad are deserting me, Pam." He'd been encouraging us to go until that moment.

66

"David, are you sure you'll be OK?" I asked, concerned, as Pam and I entered the living room.

"No. Mom, but I want you both to go. Don't worry," he added in a lighter tone.

"Okay. We'll be in daily contact, and we can come home immediately if needed. The Lord will be with you, David, don't forget," I said unnecessarily. I knew instead of David's trust in God being weakened by the auto accident, his faith seemed even stronger.

Together with Wayne I prayed aloud. "Lord, heal David completely while we're gone. Take that tiny lump off his scalp. Let me see him jumping, leaping on two strong legs. Lord, may I see his wedding some day. Please let it be so."

We packed for our trip to Orlando and the Caymans feeling like the whole world was out of control.

Early Saturday morning we were in flight to Orlando, Florida. Although our original departure day had been days earlier, a doctor's explanatory letter about the accident allowed us ticket changes without penalty. Sympathetic concern we received from airport personnel as they read the letter touched us. The kindness of other people during our times of pain never failed to amaze us.

I relaxed in the airplane as it entered the wispy layer of clouds. It seemed as though a veil now separated me from the limitations of the world and I could communicate unhindered with my Creator.

"Lord, Dave's entirely in your hands. Bless and protect him." I prayed as the plane climbed. "Flood Dave's body with the fullness of health."

Upon arrival, we went immediately to the local Professional Golfer's Association Show at the Orlando Convention Center. Our business acquaintances there knew nothing of our trauma of the last few months. I felt the relief of doing a familiar routine activity. Even though caring for David was a work of love we never minded, the daily unpredictability we faced as his caregivers was exhausting. As dusk deepened we headed our rental car for Lucerne Hospital in downtown Orlando. Only our intense desire to see David's best friend, Ricky, could get me into the unpleasant antiseptic hospital setting again.

We located Ricky's room easily. He was dozing with a scarcely eaten dinner tray in front of him. I was pleased to hear the lift in his voice as he said hello. I kissed his forehead thinking how dear Ricky was to us.

Lovable sweet Ricky was in second grade when he and Dave met; now he was a big, six-foot senior. What a privilege to be part of this child-become-man's life.

My joy was dampened by the sight of his pale, post-surgical appearance. We'd learned from his parents he had his spleen removed that morning. His nurse bustled in and explained to us that Rick was doing well, but needed to eat more.

Rick asked the nurse politely, "May I have another pain pill, please?"

She checked her watch. "In another half hour." Then she slipped away.

"Oh God, why must he suffer, too?" I groaned inwardly. "How about a few bites, Rick?" I urged, lifting a spoonful of Jell-O from his "liquids" tray. Rick opened his mouth dutifully.

Between spoonfuls he asked, "How's Dave?"

"He got out of the hospital yesterday," I said. "'We're praying for total healing for both of you."

'You guys are really going through tough times," Wayne said.

I heard the concern in his voice.

Rick responded in a resigned tone, "I had my spleen removed today," as if he was now an incomplete person.

"'We know - that's O.K. - you can manage fine without it, really."

I continued to feed Rick. After a couple more spoonfuls, Rick held up his hand and insisted, "No more."

Removing the tray I asked, "Would you like a cool washcloth for your head?" I wanted to do something, anything for him.

"Sure," Rick said faintly.

"Bless him Lord," I prayed silently as I placed the cool compress on Rick's forehead. "Why should these fine young men be afflicted?"

Rick's parents, Shirley and Biff, arrived and gave us big hugs. We chatted in Rick's room until the nurse brought more pain medication and Rick slipped into a deep sleep. Then we moved to an outdoor visitor's deck. Under the beauty of twinkling stars on a magnificent warm winter evening in Florida, we talked about the ugly enemy that had attacked our children.

Biff said, "I've asked myself over and over, what happened?"

We shared our mutual experiences and tried unsuccessfully to pinpoint what might have caused their cancer. To our original bond of friendship, we added this even stronger bond of fighting for the lives of our sons.

Promising to keep in telephone contact and prayer, we left and headed our rental car toward Miami.

Before falling asleep in our motel room, I thanked God that Rick's form of lymph gland cancer, Hodgkin's, had a good success rate. Fortunately it had been caught early. I wished I could say the same for David.

Following a tearful reunion in the Miami airport with our dear friends, the McLuens from Georgia, we all boarded the plane to the Caymans. For the next six days we were surrounded by the azure blue waters of this island paradise. We had blessed times of prayer and praise, morning and night, in our friends Chuck and April's oceanfront condo.

While on the islands we attended three prayer services with a miracle-witnessing Christian community. Twice the entire community gathered around Wayne and me and prayed specifically for David's healing from cancer, even that his broken leg would heal miraculously.

On one occasion a tall, thin native man concluded the prayer in a loud, resonant voice prophesizing, "Yet shall he live!

"Amen." I felt a shiver of anticipation go through my body as he spoke.

While laughing and crying with our Christian friends some of the heaviness of the last few months was lifted. Most importantly, we were renewed and "prayed up" for what was ahead.

Every night we'd placed the slow laborious call from the Islands to home and were reassured that David was okay. On our departure day we were anxious to get back to check David's progress, after all the prayers said on his behalf. We had high hopes of seeing a miraculous healing in our son. Little did we know the shock awaiting us.

CHAPTER 11

After a blissfully uneventful flight we entered our house eagerly. I went directly to the sofa bed with arms outstretched. "Hi David," I hugged him gently. One look and my cheerfulness faded. I saw with horror David had lumps across his forehead now. As David strained to raise himself to a sitting position, it was evident that his strength was further depleted. Perhaps sensing our shocked reaction, David turned away.

I struggled to compose myself and try to be enthusiastic. "David, while we were gone, we had powerful prayers from our old and new friends."

"Good, I need them." David's eyes were hollow.

"Tell me how you're feeling," I said, anticipating his answer.

"I hurt everywhere. My stomach feels like its being ripped apart."

My mouth went dry and I could barely speak. "I'll be right back after I say goodbye to Pam." I hurried into the kitchen, with Pam following. "Pam, why didn't you tell me on the phone?" I agonized.

"David insisted we were not interrupt your trip, besides what could you do? He refuses to see any doctor except his orthopedic surgeon for follow-up." Pam was obviously frustrated. "His next appointment is Tuesday. He's hardly moved out of bed. Because of the stomach pain, David can't eat much. I called the internist. He said David may have the flu. The hospital staff said it could be stress ulcers from all his pain following his surgeries. David refuses to talk about the lumps on his head."

"Pam, thank you." I sighed. "I know you've taken good care of David along with Jeannette and our

Grandmas and Grandpa and Frank. We still need a miracle, honey. Keep praying."

"Mom I've got half of Evanston praying for David. Some of my college friends who never prayed before in their lives have been so touched by what's happened to David that they're praying daily." We hugged sharing a womanly nurturing bond for this beloved brother and son.

That evening after David fell asleep, Wayne and I tried to console one another in our disappointment. Not only was David not healed, he was actually much worse.

"Oh God? When will You work a healing? I refused to ask the other nagging question. Will You work a healing?" I still dared to believe He would.

Day by day we watched the yellowish tinge deepen on David's skin. A strange, slightly nauseating odor began; I thought at first it was from David's cast. I soon suspected that the sickening smell was the cancer. David slept on a blanket on the family room floor. He'd become too weak to climb on and off the sofa. During the night we half slept in an adjacent room listening for his calls.

After we were back about a week, David awoke from a fitful nap sweating heavily. "Mom, I dreamt I was in a burning house and every passageway I entered filled with smoke and fire before I could get through. It was real scary. I couldn't get out."

Silently I thought, Oh David, that's like your life. What can I do for you? God show us how to keep him comfortable at least, I begged.

Unknown to David, I called his former radiologist. He recommended we bring him back for more radiation. "It won't heal him, but it might possibly alleviate his discomfort."

I also contacted the medical consultant from the University Cancer Clinic who had previously confirmed the oncologist's initial protocol. His suggestion etched in words of granite in my heart was quite simple. "Take David on a nice trip somewhere. There's really nothing we can do for him. If he stopped chemotherapy the first time, what he'd have to endure now would be so rigorous and risky it wouldn't be worth it."

"Lord," I prayed aloud, "Is this your advice, also? I just can't believe it is."

After we were back about a week, on a Wednesday night about 4 a.m., I awakened with severe pain searing my chest. My heart was palpitating rapidly. I thought I was having a heart attack. It took all my strength to call Wayne's name.

Wayne awoke immediately.

"I can't breathe!" I whispered.

Then as quickly as the sensations came, they disappeared, leaving me feeling as though a steamroller had flattened me like a roadrunner in a cartoon. Wayne held me very close and kissed me tenderly.

When I was able to speak again I said, "Wayne, I felt like I was dying, and I didn't care. Then I thought, No, not yet, not as long as David still needs me."

"Yes, and I need you too," Wayne said, stroking my hair. "It's emotionally exhausting for you caring for David alone all day. At least I get a break when I'm gone at work. You need more rest."

"It's not lack of sleep that's upsetting me most. It's that in the natural realm of reason and circumstances, we're losing this battle."

"I'm still believing God's Word for David's recovery. When I read Scripture with an open mind, and meditate on it as though for the first time, I have to agree with David's belief that Jesus will heal him. God's word is real and true, or it isn't. God can intervene at any time, but maybe He won't, until the final moment."

So David had totally persuaded Wayne.

"I'd just read a book about a minister who was healed after he was on his hospital deathbed. That could happen to David, or God could choose to take him."

Wayne took my hand gently. "Whatever we need to be ready to release David you know."

I couldn't look at Wayne. I wanted to turn away from his words, although I knew he was right. I gulped. "I know. How are you managing to hold up, darling?"

"It helps me to write my thoughts and feelings. I get so confused." Wayne went to his dresser and pulled out another worn piece of paper. He read, "It would appear that all is lost with David. His symptoms are worse and spreading fast. I praise God that David is still here with us. We are standing on God's Word and claiming a healing. I truly believe that Jesus wants David well for He is love and He healed all who came to Him and believed He would." Wayne took a deep breath and went on.

"It's hard to find words for Dave. Lord, all I can do is go back to your Word. I read, search, pray, but the answers seem to come and go. Lord speak to all of us and let us rest in your will. I gave David to you long ago and I give him to you again, Lord. I used to believe that you didn't become involved in our dally cares, but Lord you showed me different. You have blessed us repeatedly. Praise you Lord, thank you."

A little sob escaped my throat.

Wayne continued, "In the face of Dave's illness, it is hard to trust and believe, but to whatever end God leads, I will still believe His Word. I wish I knew what was blocking healing, but God's thoughts are not mine. Our faith and prayer is not simply a formula, but what we believe and I know that somehow God will honor this faith."

Wayne's voice shook as he continued, "Am I crazy, Jesus? Are not Your words for us today? But many are healed and some not, why Lord? I know we don't deserve Your goodness. We're not special, holy people, we're sinners and weak, but You still love us I know and want to give us life in abundance - the gifts of the Spirit, we are Yours and you are ours."

I looked up at Wayne as he kept reading. The tears in my own eyes matched his.

"Lord, you found me my wife, saved me in car accidents, gave me four wonderful children, loving parents and family, satisfying work that supplied all our needs. Thank you Jesus." Wayne concluded, "Can I ask for one more favor? Heal Dave! Please Lord! Thank you for listening and answering. In Jesus' name I pray, for You have said, 'Ask and you shall receive.'"

"Yes, yes, Lord." By now I was sobbing quietly. Eventually I fell into an exhausted heap in Wayne's arms.

To get a full-night rest the next night, Wayne insisted I sleep alone upstairs where I couldn't hear David. Wayne slept downstairs to be available to care for David. David had started hallucinating during the night. It had been a long time since I'd had more than a few moments alone.

I wanted to sort my own emotions to get a perspective on what was happening. David was very ill, but he still refused to see an oncologist. I couldn't accept the hopeless words of the University Clinic doctor. I slept fitfully with thoughts swirling through my head.

The next morning I tried to awaken David at 10:00 a.m.. for his orthopedic doctor's appointment by shaking him gently.

"Mom, I just can't make it. I was up most of the night in pain. Reschedule it, please." David peered at me through half-closed eyes.

"I'll try."

I came back and whispered to him a few minutes later, "The receptionist squeezed us in on Friday." As an afterthought I added, "that's three days from now, realizing how difficult it was for David to keep the days straight with his erratic sleeping.

Later that morning when David was fully awake, I said, "You know David, you really should go back to Madison." I didn't say the word oncologist, but David knew what I meant. Since receiving the letter from his former doctor, David had become so opposed to him that he almost growled when I mentioned the word "oncologist."

To my immense surprise, David agreed. However, by the next day, he was back to negative statements and firmly refused to see any doctor other than the orthopedist.

I prayed for God's intervention somehow. Maybe some new advance in cancer treatment had been discovered in the past four months. I desperately wanted to have David evaluated again: I couldn't believe all was hopeless.

Months earlier, Nancy, a nurse friend whose husband was a pediatrician, gave me the name of an oncologist in Madison, who'd treated her husband's brother successfully. His name was Dr. Love. Nancy also brought us an audiotape called "Jesus the Physician" by Bill Hybels of Willow Creek Community Church. He encouraged prayer with medical intervention as well. "In case you ever need it," she'd said. Nancy's voice quivered as she offered this information fearful of offending us. She knew we were standing in faith. I'd carefully put the card into a drawer and pulled it out now. If ever we needed to review every option, the time had come.

That afternoon I slipped upstairs, while David was napping, to call Dr. Love to ask him to see David. I felt like a criminal betraying a sacred trust; yet, I sensed this was right. Wayne had agreed. The Lord expects us to use the brains he's given us.

Dr. Love's nurse said, "Dr. Love will see David, but only after he examines David's medical records to determine whether he can be of help."

I called Dean Clinic and made arrangements for the medical transcripts to be sent to Dr. Love immediately. How we'd get David to go unless we gagged and bound him hadn't occurred to me yet.

Days later I checked back with Dean Clinic and was told the records were being held up because we hadn't signed a release.

"Why wasn't I informed of this requirement?" I demanded of the receptionist. I'd have driven to Madison or had the release federal expressed for my signature. We've lost valuable days," I said with barely controlled fury. Without even an apology, the office girl droned that she would send out the necessary form.

I sensed the battle being waged, between sickness and health, good and evil, deeper yet, God and Satan.

CHAPTER 12

On Friday, an icy cold February day, Wayne took off work to help me get David to the orthopedist. I couldn't hold David alone if he slipped. In order to walk on crutches in his weakened condition, David had to lean his weight on both of us. We struggled to get him into the car.

David was nervous and irritable about going to the appointment. We were uncomfortable with his extreme anger toward doctors knowing that God uses doctors in mighty ways. The bitterness that David expressed was not compatible with the Christian mandate of forgiveness.

The three of us must have been a weird sight tottering into the half-full orthopedist's reception room. I expected a wait, but mercifully we were shown back immediately. Perhaps the office staff realized wisely they might not get us up if we sat down. I looked up at the soft blue walls with a Saturday Evening Post Rockwell magazine cover depicting a doctor treating a child, as we helped David onto the examining table. "Lord, help Dr. Knavel help David," I prayed.

The doctor came in at once. I knew from past experience that he was an abrupt, but highly competent doctor. His skillful hands examined David's leg. When he looked up at David, Dr. Knavel asked, "When were you last seen by an oncologist?"

David hedged.

"Three months ago," I answered.

The doctor pressed on David's belly and reported, "Your spleen's enlarged." He examined the skin color inside David's hands and arms thoughtfully. Without looking at either Wayne or me, Dr. Knavel announced, "You need to be in Madison, young man. Who's your doctor?"

I chimed in, "We're in the process of switching to Dr. Love at the University of Wisconsin-Madison Clinic. David's former doctor can assist with the arrangements."

"Well, I'll call them both right now." With that Dr. Knavel strode from the room.

David spluttered, "No." He glared hatefully at us. "I'm not going and you can't make me."

I said firmly, "Yes, son, you are going because we're getting a court order to make sure you're examined." I had no idea how to do this, but a friend had suggested it as a recourse just that morning. David couldn't have been more furious if I'd slapped him. My heart ached to see his disappointment. I knew he felt we were betraying him. I couldn't think about that now.

Wayne said, "I'm sorry David. We have to be sure that we've done everything we can for you. You can still refuse treatment, but you need to know your present condition and if you have any other medical options." Wayne left the room to make some business calls.

I was alone with David in the examining room. Crude, blasphemous words spouted out of David's mouth. I'd never heard him use swear words or that guttural voice before, even through all his painful previous treatments. On top of that, David, who had been too weak to hold a cup of water, suddenly developed an amazing strength in his arms. He used his crutch like a sword lashing it back and forth at me. When I dodged his attempts, David clenched the sides of the table and tried to lift himself off. I edged out of the room feeling more shock than fright from his angry attack.

I met Wayne in the hall. "That's not our son. It's like some demonic spirit is trying to prevent David from getting help. I can't go back."

From the door I watched David's agonizing struggle to stand up and walk out. Tears ran silently down my cheeks. Thank God David was just a little too weak and the leg cast too cumbersome. I remembered the Genesis verse, "What man had done in evil, God will use for good." Finally I understood its meaning. In awe I thanked God for David's broken leg and heavy cast on his body that prevented him from walking out because he surely would have.

Dr. Knavel returned from his calls. "We're all set at the hospital."

"I noticed when we pulled up earlier there was a medical transport vehicle outside your office. Is it still there? We can't drive David in our auto in his current condition."

Dr. Knavel said, "It left, but we can call for another one."

I was incredibly grateful for his efficient, take-charge manner.

David's refusal was so adamant, we almost wavered. Out in the hall Wayne said, "Maybe we should wait until Monday because Tamara and Greg and Pam are coming in for the weekend. The hospital staff probably won't do any testing until Monday and it's already Friday afternoon."

I answered, "Darling, I believe we need to use this opportunity that God has provided now. Let's not miss it."

Twenty minutes later, two medical technicians walked in carrying a stretcher. David squeezed his lips into a thin line as they transferred his rigid body and strapped him down.

We arranged for the driver to stop at Dean Clinic on the way to pick up copies of David's previous medical records that were needed for admission to University Hospital in Madison.

David's last words to us were, "Don't do this to me. I'll never speak to you again if you do." His ice-like eyes stared straight ahead.

I bent over the stretcher. "Son, I'm so sorry." Inside I was sobbing. After telling David we'd be in contact with the hospital we said goodbye, feeling the pain of parents who must sacrifice their relationship for the potential benefit of their children's ultimate good. Nobody ever promised us life would be easy.

To God be the glory that we didn't delay. One day longer may have been too late.

Nine a.m. the next morning Dr. Richard Love called Wayne at his cross-country ski business. "You better get here right away. Your son needs an emergency procedure or he'll be dead within twenty-four hours. And he's refusing the treatment," Dr. Love added in an incredulous tone.

"The cancer spread that fast?"

The doctor's voice strained to remain patient. "We took a blood test when David arrived in ER last night. His blood is full of blasts. The normal white blood count is 4-6000. David's count is approaching 200,000 and multiplying rapidly. We need to filter them out of his blood, but he won't let us," Dr. Love snapped.

What doctor liked to have a patient decline a proven life-saving procedure, even if it's temporary?

"Dear God, no," Wayne moaned.

"At this rate David could be dead of a stroke or a heart attack at any minute. David's blood is thick with them."

"David's eighteen. He must sign for treatment."

"He says he's waiting for God to heal him and refuses treatment. We have a technician standing by for an emergency leucropheses if you get David's consent. The procedure takes a couple of hours; it's uncomfortable but not painful. At this point, it's David's only hope." Openly frustrated, Dr. Love shouted into the phone. "Perhaps you can talk some sense into him."

"We'll try," Wayne said, remembering the frozen look we last saw on David's face. We'll leave immediately, but we're an hour and a half away," Wayne said rapidly.

"That's too long," the doctor boomed, "Here's the number of David's room. Call him. See what you can do. We'll keep trying on our end ... Wayne rang me immediately. In amazement I listened to his report.

"I realized David was very sick, but not within hours of death." I felt like my own blood had stopped circulating, and darkness and light were competing for the limited air in my lungs. David's sisters and brother, Tamara, Pam and Dan, had all gathered around the kitchen table hanging on every word.

"I'll pick you up in ten minutes." Wayne ordered. "In the meantime, call David and try to talk him into this."

My fingers trembled as I dialed the number the doctor had given us. Waiting for the connection, I thought, "David could be dead before we arrived."

My call reached David's room directly. David was angry with me for authorizing his medical transport to the hospital to see an oncologist. His sisters, Tamara and Pamela, got on the extension phones. They begged David to go through with this emergency procedure. David ignored their pleas and said his goodbyes. In desperation Tamara yelled, "David, I'm going to tell everyone you're a coward." David's typical brotherly response was "Go ahead, I don't care."

I sobbed. "David, have the treatment just so we can get there and see you once more. Your birth was placenta previa. I nearly died during delivery. Now you can at least have this emergency treatment, and give us time to get there and see you one last time."

David said to his sister, Pam, on the extension, "What's the use prolonging it? I'm going to die anyway if God doesn't heal me."

Pam answered, "I can understand why you want to make this decision after all you've been through. You've been a wonderful brother. I'm going to miss you. But remember one of your favorite movies, *It's A Wonderful Life?* Everyone prayed for Jimmy Stewart and God heard their prayers."

Tamara coaxed, "The TV movie *Vital Signs* you made at work is going to be shown Monday night. If you die today, you'll never see it. At least have this treatment so you can live until Monday."

"Maybe God wants more time for your miracle and this is how He's providing it," Pam said.

David didn't answer.

Over the phone we heard the doctor come into David's room and start yelling. The doctor minced no words, using a few swear words David had never heard at home. I'm sure they weren't taught in medical school. The doctor's voice thundered, "This isn't a soap opera. This is life or death. You want God to heal you. He can still be the one who heals you, if that's what you want, but you must do what you can. We aren't treating the cancer by this, just cleaning out your blood vessels."

Pam added, "David, listen to the doctor, then you can evaluate your options clearly."

Dr. Love's voice softened in the background as he said, "Remember without this procedure right now, I give you twenty four hours or less to live. Now think about that real good."

David was back on the line. "I've got to go."

"Please David, we love you," I said. My voice trailed off into the dial tone.

I threw some overnight things into a bag before Wayne arrived and we all piled in. Inside the van I laid my head on Wayne's lap, holding it up was such an effort. "We talked to David, his answer is no." I prayed silently as we drove to Madison not knowing if we'd find David alive or dead.

The ride seemed interminable, but at last the large University Hospital Complex loomed before us.

We parked and ran to the Hematology floor asking directions along the way. When we found the room we'd been told was David's, it was empty. An aide was making up the bed.

"Oh, no, we're too late," I moaned.

The startled aide looked up wide-eyed and said, "If you're looking for David Rolfs, he's been moved to another wing for leucropheses. I'll show you the way."

Thank you, Jesus. My heart soared as we followed her toward David's treatment room.

David was lying with arms extended crucifixion style on an elevated hospital bed with one-quarter-inch tubes stuck into his elbow joints. A mass of whirring machinery seemed to fill half the room. David's blood was surging through the maze of tubes.

David looked up at me with angry, cold eyes, and then turned his gaze toward the wall.

I watched transfixed as David's blood was pulled from one vein, spun through the machine and then returned through his other vein. I remembered Abraham's preparation to sacrifice Isaac. God are you saying, "Trust and obey to the ultimate degree whatever we see?"

I said nothing. Words of comfort weren't appropriate yet.

But I felt a tiny warm wave of hope wash over me.

David's brother, sisters, and brother-in-law clustered around him. "We're so glad you agreed to this," one of them said.

David glared back. "Only this, that's all. No more chemo."

"Okay, we understand."

Kathy, the technician, said, "Just fifteen minutes before you arrived, David consented to this leucropheses treatment. I've been waiting around past the end of my shift because no one else here knows how to operate this equipment. Our other technician is in Hawaii."

"Thanks," I said, moved to tears by her eagerness to help.

Kathy smiled at David. "I'm glad I didn't waste my morning for nothing. After all David's been through, according to what I read in his chart, I can understand why he was reluctant. Plus it's got to be had to think clearly with all these blasts inside him." She added, "My husband strongly believes in God's healing powers, too."

David was exhausted after his treatment and still refused to talk to us. Although that was emotionally hard, we weren't deeply concerned. Hopefully he'd come around eventually. If not, this was a sacrifice we'd chosen to make for his life. What parent wouldn't?

The F4/6 resident doctor came in and informed us that a meeting was scheduled with our family the next morning to discuss David's options.

God, you mean he has OPTIONS? My spirit leapt. A faraway tingle of music sounded quietly in my ear.

CHAPTER 13

Our entire family was present at the 11 a.m. meeting with three doctors Sunday including David's Grandma Rolfs and Aunt Deanna, two special people in his life. As I entered the staff room located to the left of the ward clerk's desk, I felt like I was walking on stepping stones placed by God.

After introductions, Dr. Love began. "David's stable, but only short term. We'd like to start prednisone immediately, if he'll agree, and then see if we can get him into remission again. What's with this God business? Why is he opposed to medical treatment?"

David's aunt answered, "You have to understand where David's coming from. He's a very bright young man. He's been misdiagnosed and treated unsuccessfully so many times he's lost his confidence in doctors. His odds of survival were never good anyway. Now he's placed all his trust in God."

Dr. Ershler shrugged. "Well David's a prime candidate for the bone marrow transplant procedure. In the last few months we've been having success with this experimental treatment. "

"How does the process work?" Wayne asked.

Dr. Ershler explained. "We bring a patient to the point of death by destroying their own bone marrow with massive doses of chemotherapy and TBI, total body radiation. Then we rescue him with a sibling's marrow. The only danger to the sibling is the use of general anesthesia, same risk as for any operation. The donor will be up and around in a day or two, and their body will quickly produce more marrow to make up for what's donated."

"And David?"

"The odds of living through the rigorous preparation and aftermath aren't as high as we'd like, but David's young, which gives him a better chance. You have three other children, and one of them could be a good match. It's certainly worth a try. I believe he can make it."

We listened enrapt. We'd heard the phrase, bone marrow transplant, once or twice before as a far-out experimental procedure, but never as an option for David. Deep down, I too believed this could work. But would one of us be a good match, Lord?

"Once we start this procedure, there's no stopping midcourse and turning back," Dr. Love said firmly.

The doctors wanted more information about David's previous medical complications. They asked about his belief in God. "Is this lifelong or newly acquired foxhole religion?"

"David seriously believes God can heal him. But you also need to understand what his medical experience has been like."

Wayne explained the many misdiagnoses and the unexplainable treatment complications. "David intensified his belief in God as his only option since he lost faith in the medical profession."

"However, David had confidence in his orthopedic surgeon who put the cast on his leg after the accident a month ago." I added.

"David's attitude makes sense based on what he's been through," Dr. Ershler said.

"We understand his disillusionment. We're not God, much as we'd like to be," Dr. Love said. "But what do you believe?"

I guessed the doctor was sizing us up to see if we would be a detriment to David's advancing through treatment.

Wayne said, "We believe God heals through natural and supernatural means. God has placed within man the ability to develop lifesaving medical procedures. It's foolish not to use any viable medical means available to us."

After we explained the details of David's previous spinal chemo problem, the staff doctor said, "We may be able to find a way around that problem. The first step is getting David to agree to be treated. Then we need to try for remission. We're not exactly sure why, but this procedure works best on patients who are in remission. Since David hasn't seen massive chemo, I think he can achieve remission again." Dr. Ershler's sincere assurance was contagious.

"Then what?"

"The bone marrow procedure requires about two months of continuous hospitalization. Then David will have a whole new blood system. Technically we don't even use the word remission, we think of this as healing. There's no lengthy protocol, which should appeal to David. You either make it or you don't."

I looked around the room wanting to make sure I wasn't dreaming.

"Now all we have to do is convince David. He still refuses treatment, but we'll give him a little time. Getting those blasts out of his bloodstream will help him think more clearly and feel a little better. Living may seem attractive again. At least we've got some leeway now," Dr. Love said with relief.

"I'm going to present it to David now," Dr. Ershler said rising. I floated out of the room filled with the euphoria of new hope. It was short-lived.

Out in the hall we asked a nurse about bone marrow transplant.

"It's like a trip to hell and back." She described the horrors of it.

Later that afternoon, the hospital chaplain made his rounds. Wayne and I asked his opinion of the transplant procedure.

The chaplain shook his head. "They never work. I have a doctor friend, a prominent and highly respected neurosurgeon, who had an autologous transplant about two months ago. He's home now in isolation. Come with me and I'll call him and you can question him yourself." Before I could respond he led me to an empty social worker's office and made the call.

The pleasant male voice of Dr. Geickert said, "I'm delighted to offer help." He described his autologous transplant at Johns Hopkins Hospital in Maryland. In autologous transplants the patient's own bone marrow is removed, purified of cancer cells, and then returned to his body. They were not then performed at the University of Wisconsin- Madison.

Dr. Geickert asked about David's previous treatment.

I told him about the excruciatingly painful spinal complications.

"It sounds like your son developed chemical meningitis from the injections. Perhaps this can be avoided by using a steroid injection prior to the chemo."

Whew! A big concern of several months ago tossed off with an expert explanation.

Dr. Geickert continued, "If your son decides to have the transplant, which I strongly recommend because it's his only hope, have his oncologist call me, and I'll explain the preventive procedure in detail."

"Thank you, doctor. I can't tell you how I appreciate your expertise and encouragement! David must make the final decision, but he wants to consider all the facts. You've helped us decide what counsel to give him."

"Good luck," he said.

I replaced the receiver slowly, overwhelmed with this incredible incidence of God's intervention. (Later we sadly learned Dr. Geickert died of complications from his transplant.)

"Thank you." I beamed at the surprised chaplain standing at my side and hurried to share the good news with Wayne and David. Although David still wouldn't speak to me, he didn't object when I entered his hospital room. I continued to make one-sided conversation. I sensed David was struggling with his desire to have me near and his anger that I allowed his orthopedic doctor to send him here by ambulance.

"David," I said, trying to control my excitement, "Not only does a doctor who's personally been through a transplant recommend it, he's also quite confident he knows how to solve the spinal chemotherapy problem." This was important, because David would need about five spinal injections.

David made no reply, but I could tell he was listening. And so Wayne and I came to believe that a bone marrow transplant was indeed God's method for David's healing. David wasn't totally convinced yet, however.

A pretty Christian nurse was coincidentally assigned to David's care. She had a tolerant spirit and a delightful sense of humor that brought the first smiles to David's face at the UW-Madison Hospital. Between taking his temperature and pulse she and David had theological discussions about the nature of God and the healing gifts of doctors.

Our family members took turns using their own unique powers of persuasion. David needed time. Yes, Lord, time - time to live, please.

Near evening I walked into David's room and found a bald, masked female patient sitting with him. His nurse, with stethoscope around her neck, was taking David's blood pressure. The nurse introduced the thirtyish woman. "This is Penny, Mrs. Rolfs, she's a Christian woman who comes here every few weeks for preventive cherno to maintain her remission."

"It's nice to meet you, Penny. Thanks for coming in to visit." Another angel to David's rescue?

David listened to her intently. Without being pushy, with a gentle power, Penny made a chink in the no-treatment shield David had forged of pain, anger and perhaps fear too.

The next day the siege of family and friends continued.

Word had spread to Delavan that David was in University Hospital lingering between life and death and refusing further treatment. Twenty-one people, friends and family, young, and old, visited David on Monday alone. They coaxed him to further treatment. Because David had still only agreed to temporary life saving measures, the blasts in his blood were again multiplying rapidly.

Peter, our minister friend, and some elders from Peter's church arrived to pray with Dave and encourage him. Peter pointed out that David's behavior toward his parents was wrong, and David needed to forgive us and ask our forgiveness.

David's small TV movie part in Ed Asner's "Vital Signs," was finally being shown for the first time after numerous delays.

Monday night we celebrated David's "stardom." We brought popcorn to his room and gathered together to watch "Vital Signs". The nurses had the movie on in their break room.

If you blinked at the wrong time you missed seeing David rowing a boat in the background. As excited as he was, David struggled to stay awake. We were all exhilarated with God's goodness in providing this interlude.

Many friends watching the movie back home in Walworth County had no idea that David was in the hospital again with cancer.

The day after the movie Scott, David's best friend, visited. He said to me respectfully, "Mrs. Rolfs, I think I need to be alone with my friend." I heard him as I was leaving the room, "Dave, you've got to try this transplant."

Little, by little, as David started to feel better, the tension between us disappeared.

Greg, David's brother-in-law, called the authors of some of the healing books David had read, and asked them to recommend David submit to medical treatment along with trusting in God. They assured David that divine healing wasn't a mutually exclusive process. God and medicine could work together.

All our family, and compassionate, confident Dr. Ershler, encouraged David with kindness and patience.

Ersh, as he asked to be called, said to David, "If it were me, I might make the same choices thus far that you have. I don't know."

David pulled himself to an upright position in the hospital bed and listened intently as the doctor continued. "But I believe we can get you in remission again and successfully perform the bone marrow transplant."

Dr. Ershler made it sound as easy as a trip to the local ice cream shop. "One of your family members can give you new marrow. Then you won't have to worry about cancer ever again. You'll have a whole new blood system. There's a boy your age being transplanted right now, and another one coming in next week."

There they were again, those precious ringlets of hope.

The doctor continued, "The bottom line is, David, this is still your decision. Either you try bone marrow transplant or you go home and die."

I shuddered. I could watch him die before, when I thought there was no hope, but not now since God presented another alternative. Not if there was even a slight chance.

"Thank you gracious, heavenly Father. Thank you for your patience, Dr. Ershler. Thank you for your bluntness Dr. Love," I whispered quietly. "Thanks to David's orthopedist for seeing the magnitude of the problem. Thanks to David's first oncologist who was cooperative in every way with getting his records prepared. Thanks to Kathy and Dr. Geickert." It was a combination made in heaven, I was sure.

The words of family, friends, and strangers spoke to David's heart - not immediately, but within the week.

"Okay, I'll try it." David announced after five days of indecision, "Let's see if I can get into remission."

Then, if only one of us would be a "perfect match."

CHAPTER 14

Remission was a big "if."

There was no guarantee. In fact, David's previous chemotherapy lessened the chances. Cancer cells became resistant to repeated chemical treatment. Still Dr. Ershler was optimistic and we believed God could do anything.

"First, we'll surgically implant a Raaf catheter into the vein near your heart," Dr. Ershler told David. "The Raaf has two ports so two products can be transfused simultaneously into your body," he explained.

"Is this absolutely necessary?" Wayne asked.

"Yes. The veins in David's arms won't hold up with all the infusions of chemicals, blood, and nutritional supplements he needs."

David became used to this new invasion in his body. He lay quietly in bed with his radio within reach. His face was pocked with the recent scars from the lymphoblastic leukemia. Stoically he received the various chemotherapy agents.

David recorded medical conversations on his tape recorder to better understand what was being done to him along with possible damaging side effects the doctors described. As scary as it was, this knowledge helped David have a sense of participation and control.

One afternoon Dr. Love pulled me aside outside David's room and said kindly, "Your son views things intellectually. He's trying to make sense out of sickness and suffering which is incomprehensible in the first place."

"You're right," I said. "This is a spiritual problem as well to him."

"When David's up to it, I'll take him back to my research laboratory and show him our work. I think that will help."

"Thank you." My eyes shone with gratitude to this doctor who got the ball rolling on David's behalf.

Ten days later we heard the coveted word after round one of chemotherapy ended. Wayne and I sat in smooth vinyl chairs at the foot of David's hospital bed. The moment froze like a picture frame in our minds.

Dr. Ershler walked briskly into David's room. "David, you're in remission! That's a big hurdle behind us." He went on. "Maintenance chemo will be needed every couple of weeks as a safeguard until you can be transplanted. We'll have time before your name comes up on the list for patients' transplants. This will give you a chance to regain the strength you lost from the car accident."

"Will I have to wait very long?"

"I hope not," the doctor answered. "I placed your name near the top of the list. We select on a priority basis, depending on the aggressiveness of the type of cancer. "With T-Cell, we can't wait long."

He explained that there were only a few beds for transplant patients at the University Hospital. The nurses gave extra care to transplant patients by checking their skin frequently, swabbing their mouths, and hooking up the endless stream of blood product transfusions and liquid nutritional supplements. "Patients can't eat for six to eight weeks after bone marrow transplant preparatory radiation because of temporary damage to the digestive tract."

"Can they survive that long without food?" I asked.

"We can now feed a person long term safely, even adding dally vitamins to their total nutrition mixtures, " the doctor said.

I asked for additional Vitamin C for its infection-fighting capability and Vitamin E, A, and B to enhance David's immune function. Ultimately, the doctors would only agree to the Vitamin C, but I appreciated that.

Rooms with special filters maintained the germ-free environment that could spell the difference between life and death for transplant patients without any infection-fighting ability.

"You can check out the University Hospital in Minnesota. You may be able to get in there sooner. They've done more transplants than we have."

David would wait the interim weeks at home. We felt jubilant walking out of the hospital with David, even if this was only a beginning. He was still on his ever-present crutches dragging his casted leg.

"My Lord and my God," I shivered in awe remembering the circumstances of our first trip here.

The next week we traveled to the University Hospital in Minneapolis, Minnesota and evaluated their transplant program. A new hospital was under construction with a separate transplant wing. However, patients being transplanted immediately would have to be switched in the midst of their recovery when their immune system was non-existent. That could be dangerous. David choose U. W. Madison.

Because of the car accident and David's cast up to his hip, he hadn't returned to college for the second semester. He spent his waiting days on the computer, watching TV, reading, and visiting friends and family by phone.

It was a pleasant, if brief lull.

An unspoken appreciation of each new day existed on all our parts. We never quarreled over mundane details of life.

When friends shared the mishaps of their day, they'd catch themselves and apologize. "But compared to what you're going through, my little problem is nothing." I'd assure them, "Everybody's problems are important, please go on ... "

But for myself I knew, unless it's a life or death issue, I have no problem at all. What's a car that won't start or a financial loss in comparison?

On an overcast Sunday, when the living-room-sized hospital outpatient lab was normally closed, Wayne and I, Pam and Dan trekked in for our private blood tests.

These would check the fine markers of tissue differentiation that could signal a match with David, and identify one of us as a donor. It was much more sophisticated testing than blood typing.

A cheerful, competent technician selected large vials for the blood that had to be drawn.

Wayne went first. He pretended to pass out when he saw the size of the needle. We all laughed a little nervously, except ashen-faced thirteen-year-old Dan. There was nothing funny about this to our youngest son. He dreaded every year his annual physical and routine blood work. Yet Dan eagerly offered to go second and stretched out his arm, shutting his eyes.

The next day Tamara had her blood drawn in a suburb of Detroit, and sent by overnight mall to Madison. All testing had to be at the same lab for standardization. There could be no mistakes. Unfortunately, the vial broke in transport. Poor Tamara had to go back in for a second blood test and she hated the process almost as much as Dan.

If only one of us could be a match! Despite Dr. Ershler's confidence we'd heard of other families with as many as six children in which none were a match for their child with leukemia. We hoped, prayed and made guesses as to who would be the chosen one. I picked Tamara or myself. I thought our personalities and coloring were the most like David's. Perhaps our blood was too.

When the results were in Tamara's blood was as close a match as could be. The only thing more perfect would have been for her to be a boy.

We chose to tell Tamara in person when she arrived for a weekend visit.

She and David were sitting and talking on the sofa in our living room.

"Tamara, we got the news. We know who the donor will be," I said with a mischievous grin. Her vibrant eyes zeroed in on me. "Who?"

Wayne and I said together, "You."

"You're joking!"

Wayne said, "No, really, Tam, it's you."

With that she collapsed sideways on the sofa, and started laughing. "Tell me it's not true."

David laughed with her.

I whipped out my camera. "Wait. I have to record this moment for posterity. Rolfs family history is being made."

She and David hugged. "I suppose you'll want to buy me some expensive jewelry as a gift for my bone marrow, David."

"Guess again," he answered. Yet, his eyes were bright with thanks.

Smiling, I said, "Tam, tell the truth, if you had to, you'd pay to give David your bone marrow. Why, I believe you'd walk all the way from Michigan to Wisconsin to do it."

She didn't deny it.

CHAPTER 15

We numbered the days prior to transplant T-day minus 7 and counting. Seven days of lethal chemotherapy and radiation; then the rescue with Tamara's healthy marrow.

"David's week of Creation," I called it, but deep within I trembled.

His last full day at home David, Dan, and I had lunch at Popeye's Restaurant in Lake Geneva. We were off the macrobiotic diet although we still tried to make healthful food choices.

While we waited for our table, David and Dan had bought a book of jokes at the restaurant gift shop. Now we laughed as David read them aloud.

"Yes, let us laugh today, Lord," I prayed silently. "And let us be able to laugh tomorrow, too, and in the days that lie ahead."

We returned home reluctantly, and helped David finish packing.

The next morning I went up to David's bedroom to get his suitcases to load the car. David was dragging himself around slowly gathering the possessions that would be his reminders of the real world for the next few months.

"Ready?" I asked, wondering how do you measure readiness of mind and heart? How do you prepare to leave when you know you may never return?

"Almost," he answered.

I saw a stack of hand-made signs. "What are these?"

"Motivational signs I made to help get me through the post-transplant ordeal."

I picked one up and read, "Get up you lazy bum!" Others said: "Rinse your mouth, NOW!" and "EAT!!!!!!!!"

On a calendar David had highlighted two months. He pointed to a circled date. "This is when I hope to be out. I also recorded a tape of my favorite music and one of bossy messages like, 'Keep going no matter what!'" David said, matter-of-factly.

"That's great." I said looking at a sign that said, "Rolfs, Delavan is counting on you."

He finished packing more methodically than usual, probably to delay departure.

Finally, we were done. "Okay, let's go, son."

After assisting David into the passenger seat, I tossed his crutches in the back. When we pulled out of the drive I noticed David looking back.

"Dave, I can guess you're thinking will I ever see my home again?'"

"Right, Mom."

"Well, I believe you will, and in record time," I said optimistically.

David smiled a little, leaned his head back against the seat, and shortly fell asleep. All the preparation had worn him out.

I was grateful for the quiet time in which to pray. Just before we pulled into the hospital lot, David awoke and kidded, "Just keep driving by, Mom."

I smiled wistfully. How I wished we could.

It seemed like there should be some hoopla to announce our arrival. Instead the hospital was winding down for the day. I reminded myself that, though momentous for us, cancer was routine at U. W. Madison Hospital.

After numerous trips up the elevator and down the halls with baggage, I was ready to help David settle in. First I scoured every inch of the room with the Lysol solution I'd brought, spraying the telephone, even the doorknobs with disinfectant. There was no way any infectious germs were getting into my son's body after the transplant destroyed his immune system. Then we arranged David's personal items to make the room seem as homey as possible. I hung a big picture of a cat. David's favorite animal. David posted his motivational signs and family pictures around the room. I arranged silk flowers. Real ones were forbidden because of their potential to cause infection.

"David, where shall I put this?"

It was a poster-size picture of David and Tamara dressed in guerilla warfare outfits on a simulated cover of Time magazine. The picture was taken at Great America the previous summer. The caption read appropriately: "A man for the 80's". It was April 1985.

"Set it on the window sill, so I can see it when I look outside," David requested.

Moving back to see if it was straight, I said softly, David, you're definitely that. A man who can adapt flexibly to ever-changing circumstances and find tranquility within your inner self. You've experienced deep, fearful pain without being broken by it. Although you love activity and prize your friends, I know you can survive this isolation."

"I can always depend on you to be in my fan club," David answered modestly. Our communication had returned to its easy banter.

In the meantime, medical technicians scurried in and out doing evaluative procedures on David. After awhile, a young doctor came in and sat down on the edge of David's bed. He looked at David, then me, before saying bluntly, "David has a problem with his heart. We may not be able to do the transplant."

"His heart?" This was a whole new issue no one had ever mentioned. "Is there danger of an imminent heart attack?"

"No. Nothing like that."

In the next breath he added, "I'm discharging David until we can evaluate his condition more thoroughly. I sincerely regret having to give you this news, but our tests indicate his heart isn't strong enough to go through this."

David and I simultaneously looked at each other then around the room at all the items in place. The doctor's gaze followed ours.

"I'm sorry, you'll have to repack everything. We can't leave your belongings in here if you're not a patient," he said.

I moaned audibly.

The doctor added more kindly, "You can leave everything in a staff room until we've made a final decision. Just box it up and the nurse will find a safe place." He patted David on the shoulder and was gone.

David slumped on the bed. I stood in a motionless stupor for a few seconds. Then I began to silently repack David's possessions and fill his overnight bag for home.

I prayed silently. Lord. Lord! What next? Is this it? Is the transplant to be over before it begins? A chance for life, beckoning, and within reach, and now gone again.

I called Wayne to explain the latest development, "Don't drive here after work, because we'll be on our way home."

David mumbled bitterly, "Tell Dad I'm a reject."

We remained silent on the drive back, trying to blot this incomprehensible happening from our mind. He was so prepared, I thought angrily.

Doctor Ershler called Saturday and said matter-of factly, "David's cardiac function won't interfere with the transplant. It's not uncommon for heart damage to appear after chemotherapy, but, in time, most of it is corrected. We'll decrease the chemotherapy that we'd normally use, as a precaution, but we're confident we can still give enough to eradicate his marrow. I've rescheduled David for next week."

I was tempted to reply, "All this upset for nothing!" Instead I said, "I'll tell David the news."

On Thursday and Friday, David received the initial chemotherapy to prepare for transplant. His doctor gave him permission to go home for the weekend to be with us.

David's spirits were obviously lowered by the delay in starting and Dr. Ershler's simple explanation hadn't perked him up.

Sunday night came all too soon. After dinner Wayne suggested our family go to the local Dairy Queen called Anchor Inn. As we sat on a picnic bench eating sundaes, Wayne's expression became serious. "I wanted you together to tell you something. I believe David is going to be healed."

We all looked at him strangely.

"C'mon Dad what do you mean? You've only said that a hundred times before." David brushed the words off.

"No. This is different," Wayne insisted. "I believe God has told me you'll be healed."

Wayne had never before had an experience of hearing God's intention directly, but he was insistent.

David responded without much conviction. "Dad, I'm glad you think so. Now, can we go home?"

Wayne brought the subject up again when he and I were alone.

"It's the strangest thing, but I've had this assurance. I know it's real, because I've wanted to be confident before, but I couldn't. When I woke up this morning I had this inner peace that David will be healed."

"I'm excited to hear you say it," I said, "but I'm still scared."

Wayne drove David to the hospital the next day for the beginning of his massive radiation and extended hospitalization. David's eyes widened with terror when he was put into the room of the previous transplant patient we'd met, available only because the young man had died over the weekend. A second young man recently transplanted had just been put into intensive care due to complications from his transplant. David paced the floor in agitation. His firm resolution to proceed had disappeared. Wayne called me from the hospital to tell me David was having second thoughts. I prayed frantically that somehow the situation would be resolved and a peace settled over me.

David said, "Why bother to start? I'm going to die anyway. At least I could enjoy my last months. The patient Scott just died in this room."

The timing was terrible. Was this Satan's twisting of events? David headed for the door. "Let's get out of here."

Wayne said wisely, "Let's not make a hasty decision. We'll go to the sunroom and talk this over, okay?"

David dragged himself down the hall ignoring the pleasantries of personnel he passed. Once in the sunroom, he slumped onto a sofa and succumbed to tears of frustration.

"Dad, what's the use?"

"It's just a matter of time, David. You're going to be fine, son. I know, God has assured me."

"Yeah. Yeah," David answered without conviction. Eventually, Wayne ran out of encouraging words for David. How many times can you say the same thing, and make it sound believable? Wayne understood David's sudden depression. What basis did he have for hope? The previous transplant patient, his new friend

Scott, died almost before his eyes. How could David be persuaded his room was not a death chamber?

Wayne and David listened to the clang of lunch trays being put on aluminum racks in the corridor.

Wayne started praying silently. *Lord I need your help. What can I do or say? Please, Lord, help us.*

Suddenly a call came over the PA system, "David Rolfs, please return to your room. Someone is here to see you."

David said, "It's probably a doctor looking for me. I don't want to go. What do I tell him?"

"It's your choice, of course, but remember, I believe you can make it through." Wayne stood up. "We may as well get this over with, let's go back, David."

"I don't know. It seems so useless. I gave my word that once underway I wouldn't stop. This is my last chance to get out," David said as he hobbled down the hall on his crutches.

Instead of a doctor, a businessman whom neither David nor Wayne had ever met was waiting. He introduced himself as a new resident of our hometown Delavan.

The man said, "I saw yesterday's local newspaper article about your movie and your transplant and decided to combine a visit with my business in Madison today."

David wondered, "Who is this man?" as Mike kept speaking.

"I came to encourage you to hang tough. You can lick this beast." Mike had a vibrant healthy face and spoke rapidly.

"Don't worry about a thing," he continued nonstop. "Look at me, I had Hodgkin's disease, now I'm doing great." The man's enthusiasm and insistence on the benefit of chemo fired up David's spirit. "Chemo is effective. You'll feel like heck for awhile, but that will pass."

Wayne and David listened speechless.

Mike went on. "I'll tell you what will help. Eat plenty of fresh fruit and vegetables, even when you don't feel like it, force yourself."

As Mike spoke words of inspiration, David sat up straighter, and his face began to reflect Mike's sparks of enthusiasm. Wayne stared in amazement at the transformation Mike's words were producing in David.

Surely this was not a man, but a messenger from heaven? When Mike stood to leave. Wayne shook his hand, and joked, "Are you an angel?"

Mike said, "'Frankly, first time I've been asked that."

Wayne explained David's depression at the time Mike's page came over the loudspeaker. "You know when most people visit someone in the hospital, if the patient's not in his room, they leave. I can't think of many who'd use a page," Wayne said.

Mike grinned, "That comes from having spent lots of time in hospitals myself."

He walked to the door and turned.

"Hang in there." His gaze focused on David. "I'll see you back in Delavan, keep in touch." David pumped Mike's outstretched hand. "Thanks a lot."

Without another word David started to unpack. The room was still the site of recent death, but the gentle hum of the air filter sounded more welcoming.

Wayne let out a sign of relief. "Thank you Jesus!"

I arrived later that evening ready to spend the next two months living alone in Madison at a hotel closeby to provide extra physical help and emotional support David needed. No one had ever been transplanted with a leg in a cast.

CHAPTER 16

Dust was casting it's grey shadow on the walls of David's hospital room when David awoke and said with a pleading voice, "Mom, hold me." He looked teary-eyed. The intense chemotherapy acted like a depressant on his nervous system.

I'll always remember David's heartfelt words, "I love you Mom. I don't know what I would have done without you."

Putting my arms around him, I said, "David, dear, I love you too, more than words can say. So does Dad and your brothers and sisters and many other people. Praise God for love, the power that moves this world." Smiling broadly, I added, "Why is it that you've always been so easy to love?"

A flicker of a grin crossed David's face, and he settled back on his pillow.

I started reading aloud from the joke book we'd brought.

At the same time I recorded my voice on audiotape so David could hear the jokes when he was alone. Finally David fell deeply asleep.

Tamara arrived Tuesday from Michigan to stay with me at the hotel until her operation. The hospital required that the donor be within an hour of David's location once the eradication chemo began in case of a problem requiring early transplant.

"At last, my comrade has come." David greeted her with a smile.

Tamara and I received permission to take David on a car ride, as long as we were back in time for David's evening radiation and Tamara's pre-op exam. We drove to a little lake near the Madison Zoo.

"David, we came prepared," I said, pulling a chaise lounge pad from my trunk while Tamara spread a hospital blanket on the grass. We slathered on sunscreen and basked in the refreshing breeze. Being in restorative, peaceful nature was delightful.

As we reclined on the beach surrounded by gorgeous mallards, I said, "How I wish I always followed my inner longings and nudges, so that the Holy Spirit could operate more freely in my life. I hope you two will remain free of the silly demands we impose on our own lives."

"Mom's philosophizing again." Tamara winced dramatically. "Ignore her."

"David, your illness reinforced the importance of maintaining inner harmony."

As the sun started its descent, we reluctantly bid the ducks adieu. David lingered for a last gaze at the lake, then swung his casted leg into the car.

We returned to the hospital for Tamara's physical.

Despite an outer facade of silliness, our daughter was obviously concerned about her operation. She made inane comments to the young resident during her pre-surgical exam, while the doctor explained her operation in detail.

"The actual bright red marrow is taken teaspoon by teaspoon from your rear hip bones. The procedure lasts a couple hours. You'll feel no pain."

"Thank goodness! By the way I'd like Barbara Streisand's song, 'Second Hand Rose,' to play during surgery. That'll be symbolic of my used marrow. And I need a Snoopy blanket!" Tamara joked.

"Sure. We'll have a complete orchestra in the operating room if you like. Any other special requests, let us know," the resident bantered back.

Later, the chief transplant doctor, Dr. Hong, stuck his head in. He didn't share my belief in the benefits of

Vitamin C. I laughed when he jokingly suggested I make a paste of the vitamin to spread on Tamara and David's bodies.

My mom and dad had encouraged me to find humor in everyone and everything including myself. The children picked up on this trait, too.

"Jesus. Continue to help us!" I prayed.

Two more days until transplant! Time seemed interminable during this preparatory chemotherapy and radiation. David's former roommate, an older man named Ted, came in for follow-up treatment and died, as did the only son of two other loving parents we met. All around us, people dealt with chemo, life and death. Why, God? We focused on treasuring every day; realizing each could be our last. Patients sometimes died during preparatory BMT treatment.

"Dear God," I prayed, "how I wish I knew how to stop the slaughter of human beings by this cursed cancer. What is the secret to overcoming this horror? The only treatment with notable success involves burning and poisoning. How may we help rid the world of this scourge of cancer?"

The radiation ravished David's body's strength. He often was asleep for the night by seven. I spent the evenings sitting next to his bed reading and praying. The room had the aura of the sacred presence of God, and angels, visible and invisible. I was sure they were present.

One night as the darkness descended I went outdoors briefly and ran across the nearby track field. I visualized David with two strong legs running, and prayed that someday it would be so.

Twenty-four more hours to transplant day, May 2nd, which happened to be the National Day of Prayer.

I wheeled David's chair to the basement lab for his final radiation treatment. He was too exhausted to walk on crutches more than a few feet. My prayers had intensified because of the increased accumulation of chemo and radiation in his body.

"Lord, let only remaining cancer cells and David's bone marrow be eradicated. Protect his other organs," I prayed fervently. After each radiation session, David vomited off and on continually. During the morning his demeanor was extremely quiet. In the afternoon, words burst out in an energy surge prior to the draining p.m. final radiation.

The last night in the radiation wing, I found a gorgeous blonde, life-size doll in the children's waiting room and set the doll on the arm of David's wheelchair.

"David, your girlfriend has arrived to keep you company," I announced.

David shot me a weak grin and pushed the doll away, while the x-ray technicians laughed. "Tomorrow's the day. Aren't you excited?"

He nodded solemnly. "The rest is up to God." He rolled his body into bed exhausted. Wayne drove up after work at ten. Our marital love flourished despite the little time we had together. Because our child was threatened we felt even more strongly the preciousness of each other. We said the Our Father together, as we did each and every night whether at home or in the hospital, meditating on every word, as we spoke. Wayne prayed, "Father, David is your son too. He was yours before he was ours. Deliver him from this evil for thine is the power and the glory forever."

Tamara stayed with David while Wayne and I drove back to Delavan for a prayer service at St. Andrew's of about fifty people organized by Bob Drefs and our other Christian friends. Cursillo friends came from Milwaukee and Racine, too. We had a precious time of prayer and sharing.

These people and many more dear friends and family members were responsible for the daily messages, prayers, gifts, and calls that David received. I always expected it was this beautiful in the community of God. The kingdom truly does begin on earth. How awestruck we were at the generosity of people who loved freely in thought and deed with no holding back.

God, help us, to love and live like this for others too. The message never changed. "We'll be there to support you. Life is worth going for no matter how hard or how long you have to fight." And it was a hard fight.

I knew David wouldn't quit. Because he's one of the blessed ones Adele Rogers St. Johns speaks of in her book *Some are Born Great*. He had the ability to pick himself up when knocked down, no matter how many times and come out a victor. But this time was the hardest, and certainly David knew that Jesus' strength must be his power now.

Finally May 2nd, transplant day arrived. People across the country were praying on this National Day of Prayer in America. A team of photographers chose this day to cross the United States snapping pictures for their epic book, A Day in the Life of America. And our family's history would be affected forever by the events of this day.

Wayne and I entered David's room. "It seems like any other hospital day except that it's your birthday," Wayne said, "the day of new creation. You know, God performed the first transplant when he created Eve from Adam's rib."

"Tamara's ready for her marrow to be extracted by Dr. Hong and his assistant on the transplant team," I added.

"I know," David pretended annoyance. "She was in here at 6 a.m. waking me up to tell me."

Wayne smiled. "We'll be back later. We want to accompany Tamara into surgery."

We joined her husband, Greg, our son, Dan and our daughter, Pam who had both taken the day off to be present. "She just went in," Greg announced.

I paced the corridor and prayed anxiously during Tamara's surgery. "Lord, now two of our children's lives are at stake. Guide the doctor's hands, let there be no complications."

Finally the surgeon emerged. "Your daughter is in recovery and doing fine."

Relieved, we returned to David's room. He was sleeping peacefully. His early rising, along with the previous week of radiation had depleted his limited energy. We settled down to wait. After what seemed an eternity, Dr. Hong entered the room cradling two plastic bags filled with bright red marrow.

"I'm personally supervising this," Dr. Hong said in an almost reverential tone. He cleared a space on David's bed table, and noticing the Bible placed there said, "Maybe we ought to leave that where it is." He winked.

"You're right about that," Pam answered.

My eyes were fixed on the gorgeous red treasure Dr. Hong held. "So that's how it looks! It's the most beautiful shade of red I've ever seen!" I exclaimed.

David began to stir. "How's Tamara?" he asked groggily. Dr. Hong answered. "Everything went well. We've given her a transfusion of her own blood that we collected earlier. That will compensate for the marrow we took. She's in a post-op recovery room."

When David saw the marrow he smiled weakly. "I'm so grateful to Tam."

Dr. Hong held up one of the plastic bags like it was the Hope diamond. "We've filtered Tamara's marrow to break up any particles and irradiated it. Now we're ready to transplant this into you."

Wayne pulled out his camera, "A nice big smile everybody."

Obviously Dr. Hong was enjoying the moment with us. We watched enrapt as he tore open a two by two inch antiseptic envelope and sterilized David's chest catheter for the transfusion.

We gathered around the foot of David's bed. Wayne placed his hands on the bags of marrow and then on David's shoulders as he prayed aloud, "Lord, may this bone marrow be the source of new life and healing in David's body."

"Amen," we answered in unison.

After hanging the first bag of marrow on the IV pole, Dr. Hong released the flow and adjusted it. Tamara's marrow began to drip slowly through the tube into David's chest. Dr. Hong explained, "The bone marrow will travel immediately to one of the three manufacturing sites in David's body and begin production within two to four weeks."

It took over an hour for the life-bearing marrow to seep into David's body. We were transfixed. I murmured a prayer over and over. "God we believe in miracles. Let this be one."

CHAPTER 17

Walking into the oncology wing of the hospital each morning was like entering another world. I was never quite prepared for what awaited me behind those walls, particularly for the deaths of other patients.

The nurses never looked up as I went by. I'd become as familiar in their environment as staff and knew the scrub-up procedures by heart. I'd determined if I said one "Our Father" quite slowly as I scrubbed my hands I'd meet the required washing time. I took a fresh mask from the box in the hall each time before entering the isolation area.

At David's door I always knocked first. When I heard his quiet "Come in" I entered. My first action daily was giving him a long hug. Although he was often too weak to hug back, I could tell he appreciated the warm physical contact. I checked the room and tidied up mail and notepads. If David was having a good day, he might be sitting at the computer we'd set up in his room and playing a game.

More often, David was lying in bed receiving a transfusion or waiting for a test. Dr. Hong had shown me how to dress the sore on David's leg caused by the rubbing of his cast. Each day I unfastened the Velcro bindings of the removable cast and cleansed the ulcerated sore. I massaged the leg muscle for a few minutes when the cast was off while I prayed for perfect healing of the bones. David liked this and I was glad to be able to provide him with some physical comfort. Then I rewrapped the entire leg in gauze padding before replacing the cast.

A nurse questioned whether this task was a nurse's job, and shouldn't be performed by a visitor. But Dr. Hong felt staff was too busy to deal with the complications of the broken leg and he cleared me for the procedure.

When a nurse or doctor would come in, they watched me and waited patiently until I was done. I had to laugh. I felt so professional! Once a week the whole team of BMT doctors came to visit. David was often used as an example for teaching purposes. The chief doctor described David's condition as if he weren't present while all the interns gathered around his bed. They were all cordial, so it became a pleasant interruption to the normal cycle of a hospital week.

David lived every day with the risk of infection entering his non-resistant immune system and potentially killing him. At least six more weeks of confinement loomed before him. Days dragged by filled with the routine of waiting and praying that David's body would not reject the new marrow.

David's body had to be evaluated continually after transplant. I escorted David by wheelchair to the orthopedic clinic, ear, nose and throat clinic, eye clinic, pulmonary functions, and dental clinic. Every inch of his body was examined frequently for any sign of infection. I tried to make jokes with the clinics' staff. Usually David just sat quietly, occasionally cracking a little smile.

David and I shared Mother's Day alone at the hospital. I pushed David out to the roof deck for a sense of being in fresh sir.

David said, "Do you know how much I love you for coming here to be with me every day? I was thinking about Mother's Day and wondering what could I get you that would be special enough. I want you to take this $20 that I received as a gift, and buy yourself something."

"David, how very nice, but you keep the money."

He insisted and finally, I took the bill because it seemed so important to him. "'You're the most wonderful mother in the world," he said.

"Thank you," I replied, "but I'm sure there were ways in which I could have been a better Mom."

That evening while David slept I wrote him a letter:

"Dear Son,

The years of watching you grow into manhood – what more gift could a mom want? I remember those years of cookies and milk after school – our special time each day. Family dinners were a daily highlight, too, with lots of laughter. Memories of our Sunday evening family night when we had 'say-something-nice-about-each-other' talks and board games put smiles straight into my heart. I loved being a mother. As you children passed through each life stage I saw clearly what was of greatest value. Nurturing each of you children, unique and precious, has been an awesome privilege. And now, David, we're fighting together for your life. Where else could I possibly want to be than at your side?

Love always, Mom"

Before falling asleep in my motel room that night I prayed aloud. "Lord, the only time David doesn't throw up is when he sleeps. May he rapidly return to normal. Heal the sores in his mouth and gastrointestinal tract! Keep him strong against infection! May his blood and entire body remain cancer-free. The power is there Lord! Please release it. According to your Word, You graciously are in covenant with us not because You're some kind of glorified magician. We need You for each step and we thank you for each moment."

For more than a week, David endured constant nausea and frequent vomiting. Then a civil war began to rage within him. It started with a terrible rash over his entire body caused by the conflict between Tamara's grafted bone marrow and his host body called appropriately graft vs. host. The new bone marrow had started to attack his skin.

Other organs, the esophagus and intestines, could be attacked next unless massive doses of steroids turned the tide.

David said, "This itching on every inch of my body is worse than the strongest pain I've experienced. "Can't Dr. Hong do something for it?"

On his daily visit Dr. Hong reassured David, "You're doing normally, abnormally well. I'll prescribe antihistamines and various ointments, but there's nothing we've found that really helps. The itching comes from irritation under your skin within your body. It's a condition that develops in about 50% of patients.

"As soon as you can, I want you to eat slight amounts of food even if you can't keep it down. That will keep your digestive tract operating." David's oncologist was adamant about his eating.

I sat with David hour after hour trying to bring cheer.

The hospital days dissolved into sameness. David's room was crammed with books and some computer software, but David couldn't muster motivation or the energy to use them. One memorable day about halfway through the isolation period, the phone, precious life-link to the real world, broke the silence.

Bill Mann, a former high school friend who attended college in Madison and had visited David previously, asked if David would like to meet Dan Travanti, alias Captain Furillo, of the famous *Hill Street Blues* TV show on Sunday morning. Dan Travanti and Bill's dad and uncle involved in the University of Wisconsin alumnae reunion and could arrange it. When David hung up, his face looked like a Christmas tree. *Hill Street Blues* was one of David's favorite TV shows.

The next day Dan Travanti came through the hospital doors with the sense of presence that experienced stage and screen performers exude.

Wayne and I hurried over and introduced ourselves. "It's incredibly kind of you to come." Wayne said. "David's really excited."

"He can't quite believe it yet," I said.

"My pleasure," Dan said graciously.

"I hope you won't mind, Dan, but David's in isolation because precautions are necessary to protect him," I explained. "You'll need to scrub up and wear a mask."

"No problem," Dan Travanti replied.

With a flourish of style he scrubbed his hands and tied on a mask to enter the transplant wing.

Walking down the hall we chatted. Nurses who passed us recognized Dan Travanti and stared. What an amazing visit!

In David's room, Dan Travanti's magnetism filled every inch. Dan brought David a gift of a UW - Madison tee shirt and proceeded to autograph the back. Then he asked for a sheet of paper and wrote his personal phone number. "Call me anytime. But under no circumstances let anyone else have this number, or I'll send the Hill street squad after you!" he said with a grin.

We all laughed.

"David, when you're better, I want you and your family to come and see me in California. I'll show you around the set while we're filming. I really mean that, understand? I'll be expecting you!"

Dan Travanti said goodbye with hug and kisses for all our family. On the way out I heard him charming the nurses. The normal routine of the hospital day resumed, but the effect of Captain Furillo's visit remained with David a long time.

Dan Travanti gave David what he needed most at this precise moment - an appointment for the not-too-distant future that David wanted to keep. "Lord, Dan Travanti, Bill Mann, his parents, aunt and uncle, these people seem like a fleet of your angels. I'm so grateful!"

Our goal became simply getting through each day and not focusing on the lengthy confinement ahead. When David's spirits dragged, I reminded him, "Look how far you've already come. We're in the last weeks of battle. Victory is in sight." But before victory came another siege.

As I drove to the hospital on Friday, May 30th after an overnight respite with the rest of our family, I was aware of the intensity of the GVH attacking David's skin. I cried my heart out, sobbing to God, "We're trusting in You." I said it over and over. It was a critical time. The GVH could go either way - begin to clear or begin to attack other organs. Finally the severity of the attack subsided.

As David lie recovering from the GVH battle in U. W. Hospital, Chernoybl hit the news! Soon the whole world became familiar with the bone marrow transplant procedure. Prior to that few had heard the term.

Two days later, Dr. Hong came into David's room and said, "Many people will be needing a bone marrow transplant. I may go to Russia to assist."

I didn't always know if he was teasing or not so I answered in a joking tone, "No way, until David is out of this hospital. Unless David goes with you in a protective bubble. You're his transplant doctor. You're not allowed to leave." I tried to sound authoritative.

Dr. Hong responded with a twinkle in his eye, and slipped away.

David was allowed out of his room for short walks and to attend physical therapy sessions daily, provided he wore his mask, and scrubbed up thoroughly the second he returned. Because of his broken leg, he needed both hands on his crutches and couldn't push the IV pole like other patients. I was his constant escort and pole pusher accompanying him to his daily physical therapy session.

"I'm sure you'd prefer a beautiful brunette," I joked one day, "but you'll have to settle for dear old Mom."

The door of the Physical Therapy room was usually closed. One day it was left half-open. My eyes searched for David among the therapists and patients working one-on one with various equipment. My heart almost stopped as I saw David in a corner trying to pedal a bicycle with his hands. How pitiful he looked.

I turned away before he saw me. Our dear son! What humbling experiences illness causes. I returned in time to push him back. In the corridor outside the workout room, I spotted David in a parade of people occupying wheelchairs awaiting escorts back to the sixth floor.

"Hi." I said with my cheeriest inflection.

Sitting in the wheelchair behind David was a man with a huge growth on his neck. I was sure David had observed this; although neither of us ever mentioned the deformed patients that we saw every day. I could see in David's eyes that he was aware of the pain all around him. Sometimes I saw confusion, sometimes fear. I, too, was incredibly frightened. I was scared out of my mind because he was my son.

Wayne and I couldn't say these things to David without adding fuel that might light fires of anger and depression. However righteous these feelings were, they wouldn't help heal him.

And so, with determined effort, we avoided focusing on the horror we could so easily succumb to. We watched David submit as he clomped along on the ever-present crutches, and hobble-hopped from bed to wheelchair day after day.

David's face was still handsome, despite the scars from the lymphoblastic lymphoma that had ravaged his blood and lymph systems.

Wayne and I felt like David the King in Scripture whose mind and heart were set upon the life of his son.

At the end of the first four weeks an unexpected new scourge appeared.

I knew something was wrong the minute I entered David's room. My greeting was lost in the groan from his pervasive pain.

Lord when will the crises end?

His nurse had followed me in, saying. "David's having intense bone pain everywhere. We've called the doctor to examine him. He'll be here shortly." She turned and left.

"Mom," David moaned piteously, "Every bone in my body hurts." He twisted and turned, like a snake, totally distraught. David's lack of composure was uncharacteristic unless he was under extreme duress.

I stood by helplessly as David struggled to find a position that would alleviate the pain. He flung himself across the hospital bed and the catheter ripped out of his chest.

I looked down with shock. A pool of blood was flowing rapidly onto the floor.

"David, don't move. I'll get help." I hurried to the nurse's station.

"David's bleeding all over. His catheter's come out." The nurse hurried to his room followed quickly by the floor resident. She re-established the IV in his chest while the doctor checked David's vitals. I noticed him carefully sidestepping the puddle of blood. Turning to me, the resident said, "I'm ordering a sedative until we can determine the source of this."

I remembered David's early symptoms of leg pain, chest pain, and jaw pain.

Oh, Lord is it starting over? Oh, God, help, please, I prayed silently.

David was poked and probed all day for an answer.

The next day Dr. Hong came into David's room to deliver the test results. "The lab discovered a magnesium deficiency in your blood. David."

"This caused all that pain?" I asked incredulous.

"Yes, we'll add magnesium to the intravenous total parenteral nutrition."

That food maintained David's life during this period. He could eat no solid food yet, due to damage to his intestinal tract. Continual nausea and diarrhea plagued him.

I was upset by David's pain and cynical response and reminded again of the need to surrender David's entire being to God's purposes.

"Lord, if he can't be whole and well and a glory to you in every aspect of his life. I do give him up."

CHAPTER 18

The experiences of each day kept us on an emotional teeter-totter. Our equilibrium depended on test tube contents and squiggly numbers on papers - the unpredictable "counts" that determined if David needed a transfusion of a blood product.

We waited expectantly for David's white blood cells to increase. Without an immune system he was extraordinarily vulnerable to disease.

Each day I climbed again the mountain of faith. I had to go to the presence of God to get a perspective beyond the present moment. Then I could toss a rope down and pull David up with me.

We were on the high end of the teeter-totter when David's discharge day arrived! Stepping off the elevator on Thursday, June 12, 1986, I sensed the festive feeling on hospital wing F4/6. This would be David's real homecoming after a couple afternoon passes and one overnight trip on his birthday a week earlier.

Jane, a pretty nurse with long brown hair, approached me with a big smile.

"What's all that?" she waved at my arms overflowing with small gifts.

"Souvenirs for the nurses and doctors to remember David by."

"As if we'd forget him!" she kidded over her shoulder as she passed by.

Another nurse friend, Sandy, bounced up. "This is great! We haven't seen a person live through transplant since February. We enter the healing profession to be lifesavers. Too often we fail. In bone marrow transplant we zap apparently well patients in remission, with lethal radiation and chemotherapy. It's not easy for us, either."

"I hadn't given much thought to that."

"Only half the patients make it through this destruction to new life," she continued, "It isn't easy. We needed David's victory too." I could only nod in response. (Note: These statistics have now increased dramatically.)

My eyes were instantly wet and a thickening momentarily constricted my throat. I'd often glimpsed the visible pain of these dear, compassionate male and female nurses who walked, sometimes ran, the corridors. Certainly this success was theirs, too.

I murmured, "We're so grateful for all you've done."

I recalled phrases from the "Thank You letter" I carried in my purse to post in the staff lounge:

"How do we thank you who have walked the long life/death road with us? With gentleness and respect, you ministered to David's body and spirit.

Night and day you were available to him. You leveled with Dave and encouraged him. At times you even felt his pain. You listened patiently to our fears and questions.

We sensed you shared our anxiety and blessedly you laughed with us too. You may have wondered and questioned his ways - our ways. But always you cared and extended total energy.

We know the mystery that 'God's banner over us is love: We have known His hands and His heart here. Were David your brother or son he could not have had better care. Sincerely, All the Rolfs."

The head nurse approached. "We're having a little party in the staff lounge before you leave. See you there. We're almost as excited as you."

I grinned like a Cheshire cat from Alice in Wonderland as I entered David's room. He was scurrying around, crutches and all, finishing packing. He stopped long enough for a quick hug.

"Good morning, son ... "

I smiled at David's doctor's costume. He'd wanted a functioning stethoscope as a birthday gift. One of his doctors procured a white jacket for him, and the kind ward clerk embroidered David's name on the pocket, exactly as it appeared on the real doctors' coats.

In the past week, David had often worn this outfit complete with a rectangular blue mask like those worn by doctors during surgery as he'd hobble through the hospital corridors on his crutches with me. I laughed at the incongruity of the sight he made.

One day an elderly, near-sighted visitor approached him, "Doctor, can you tell me how to get to the blood laboratory?"

"Sure." David enjoyed her mistake and directed her. Now David's words tumbled out, "Mom, I'm glad you were able to get the gifts. You won't miss coming here, I bet!"

A half hour later we entered the little staff room behind the ward clerk's desk. Four or five nurses had gathered. Others poked their heads in and out. They welcomed us with cheers and shouts, "Yeah for David! It's party time."

"David, you've been an encouragement to us all," said a sweet nurse as she gave David a hug.

The head nurse brought in a huge sheet cake decorated with the words, "David, We All Made It Through." She said, "We brought a farewell gift for you," and ceremoniously pulled out David's machine gun-style squirt gun that she'd confiscated weeks previously. David had been squirting anyone who opened his door, be it nurse, doctor or janitor.

Applause filled the room.

David teased, "Well, it's about time you quit playing with my gun and returned it to me."

With a tinge of sadness, I observed David's crutches leaning against his chair. At least the IV connections were gone, although the Raaf catheter remained in his chest in case he needed another transfusion.

With a mother's delight I watched our son enjoy his celebration. Together we distributed the gifts of hats and cloth bags and tee shirts to the nurses and doctors.

More laughter and a lot of hugs later, we said our farewell. Helping David into the car at the hospital entrance, I felt like I had plucked the canary from its cage.

I smiled ecstatically at the parking attendant scarcely believing the day was real. We sailed through the gate like we'd been at the hospital for an hour instead of forty-one days.

I zipped along the expressway under the crown of a glorious blue sky. I reflected aloud. "Lord, when I stand before You some day, You will not accuse me of failing to be grateful."

My soul was ready to leap with praise from my body, and prance with joy.

David's welcome home, if quieter, was no less wonderful. The previous week, while Grandma and Grandpa Rolfs visited with David for a couple days in my absence. I'd gone home to scrub the house, have the furniture and upholstery cleaned, remove the plants, and relocate the pets, all according to doctor's orders. David's sister, Pam, helped tremendously. It was exhausting, but exhilarating work for David's return. We also walked through each room of the house and prayed for God's healing Holy Spirit to permeate our home.

At each entry door I'd posted a hand-written sign, "Please DO NOT Enter without a mask. Wash your hands immediately upon entering." I placed boxes of masks by the doors and Phisohex at every sink for hand washing. We couldn't be lax now. We'd come too far.

David settled in like a perch returning to water.

Ten carefree days later, our smooth sailing came to a halt. David developed a fever. Wayne and I drove him back to the U. W. Madison emergency room in sadness and trepidation.

Again I prayed, "Dear Lord, we're frightened and frustrated. Will we ever stop calling upon you in desperation?"

After examination the ER staff doctor reassured him, "David I believe your body can fight this infection. Go home and take it easy."

Obviously David's body had not been listening. The next day the fever shot up.

We contacted Dr. Longo, who was David's transplant follow-up doctor.

"David must return immediately for extended hospitalization." Again we hurriedly drove the hour and a half to Madison.

An attendant wheeled David toward a new hospital room in the same F4/6 wing from which he'd escaped less than a week earlier. David was morose and silent.

A dear nurse friend, Jane, saw him, "Why such a downcast face and stooped carriage?" David mumbled a response.

"It's the rare transplant patient that doesn't return at least once for treatment for an infection," she assured him.

I heard David muster a casual, "Hi" to another nurse buddy he passed. He quipped sarcastically, "I missed you so much I decided to come back to see you."

Once in his room with the door closed, David became sullen. "Great, here we go again ... "

I remained silent letting him vent his angry feelings. The resident came in. After the exam he said, "You need to stay a couple weeks for IV antibiotic treatment to make sure we've got this thing knocked out of you."

David looked like he'd received a prison sentence. "David, I know this is tough," I said. "Would you like me to stick around tonight?"

"No, I don't feel like talking."

"Okay, I'll be back tomorrow, son." I hugged him and we said the Our Father aloud as we did every night. His voice was dull and lifeless.

The next day I met the doctor outside David's room. "David is terribly discouraged about being here. If he only needs IV's, could we provide this at home by hiring a nurse?" I didn't want to discuss this in front of David so as not to get his hopes up if it wasn't an option.

The doctor had another plan. "After we get this infection turned around, we'll teach you and your husband how to complete the course of antibiotics at home."

Upon hearing that good news, David's buoyant spirit returned.

By the end of the week we were home again complete with a metal pole to hang IV bags on and a refrigerator shelf stacked with bags of antibiotics.

Wayne, Pam, and I took turns keeping up the hospital schedule of 5 a.m. and 5 p.m. IV's.

My first day as unofficial and uneasy nurse, I crept into David's room in the early morning light. Looking at his trusting, sleeping body, I was overwhelmed with the sense of this new responsibility. Nervously, I opened the port on the catheter that led directly into his heart vein.

I said, "David, I'm starting your IV now; you don't have to completely wake up, just stay still."

He mumbled, "Okay."

God, help me do this right! I entreated silently.

I checked and rechecked every step of the instructions I'd written out when I watched the nurse's demonstration in the hospital.

After I hooked David up, I counted the drops going through the tube to adjust the flow precisely. Then I sat down to read and pray and watch the drip, making sure David didn't make any sudden moves.

The transfusion rate was slow and steady requiring about forty-five minutes. Next the ports had to be carefully flushed and closed to prevent infection.

Finally, it was over.

I did it! Me, who used to hold my breath when I had to examine a skinned knee, and abhorred shots, had just given my first IV transfusion. *By your grace, God! Thank you, Jesus.* By doing this twice a day, we could have David at home.

Preparing foods to entice David to eat was challenging. The radiation left a metallic taste in his mouth that remained even after his mouth sores healed. Dr. Longo was emphatic, "I don't care what he eats, as long as he eats!

I joked, goodbye macrobiotic diet, hello cinnamon-sugared toast, cantaloupe and ice cream sundaes and horror of horrors, sugar-coated cereals.

David was instructed to record his temperatures morning and evening. I administered his medications, and helped him to walk in his weakened condition on crutches. Exercise remained essential. We counted off on the calendar each of these first, critical 100 days.

The removable cast remained on David's leg. I continued to unwrap it daily, examine the skin for new sores, and treat the abrasion on his ankle with sterilized water and antibiotic ointment.

Weeks passed blessedly uneventful. David slept a great deal as his body recovered from the extensive radiation and chemotherapy it had endured.

During this time our friends held a one-hour every evening, 100- day prayer vigil at St. Andrew's Church. Bob Drefs and Ruth Kempken kept a chart to organize people into time slots. Just as they approached the 100-day mark, disaster struck.

We'd planned a weekend celebration of praise. David had invited about thirty friends to a beach party on Saturday. Wayne and I were to attend his high school reunion. Sunday we planned a Mass and buffet for all our family and friends who had faithfully prayed for David and encouraged us in countless ways. Early Saturday afternoon David began to feel sick. An hour later his temperature was 103 degrees. I called University Hospital in Madison.

"Bring him in immediately," Dr. Longo ordered.

This was also the day of Wayne's thirty-year Arlington Heights High School reunion. He'd already left to play golf with his former high school teammates with whom he'd won the state golf championship his senior year. My good friend, Sue, arrived to drive me to Illinois to meet Wayne and her husband for the reunion dinner.

I was deeply torn. David's infection could require hospitalization. Should I go sit with him or proceed with our plans?

If only there were two of me.

"Mom, I'll take David to Madison," our twenty-one year-old daughter Pam offered.

"Do you think you can manage?" My eyes welled with tears. "It's hard for me to think straight at the moment."

"Sure. David can lie down in the back seat. If you'll get his things, I'll pull the car up.

"Okay, I'll pack an overnight bag and help him down. Dr. Longo said he'll meet you in E.R Thank you, sweetheart. Hopefully he just needs a different antibiotic."

I knew David was in good hands. Pam would do whatever needed to be done.

As I was helping David into the car, David's friends, Mark and Scott, arrived to set up their sound equipment for the party. David was too ill to make small talk. He stretched out wearily on the back seat.

"I'm sorry, guys. David's ill and on his way to U.W. Hospital. I need to leave immediately also. Would you please contact the guests and tell them the party's, uh, postponed. You can call from here."

"Sure," they said with shocked voices.

CHAPTER 19

At the University of Madison Hospital the staff was waiting. David's fever was 104 degrees upon arrival and rising fast. The nurses had IV's ready to go. They flushed David's body with massive quantities of fluid and antibiotics to turn around the sepsis attacking his body.

The doctor told David's sister, Pam, "Another four hours, and he'd have been a goner for sure."

We called Pam for a report every hour. Around 9 p.m. she said, "Mom, finally the doctors think they have the infection under control, but he has to stay in the hospital under observation." I breathed with deep relief. Thank you, Lord!

The next day was our scheduled outdoor praise celebration. After discussion and prayer, Wayne and I decided to proceed with our service of thanksgiving, despite David's being hospitalized and an overcast sky threatening rain.

Wayne said wisely, "Whatever the outcome, we won't rob God of the glory and praise for all that He's already done for us."

During the liturgy, I felt like Cinderella at the ball when her fairy godmother granted her request. This life and death whirl was an unreal world in which to live. I was different too, now, because I understood the fragility of this merry-go-round.

Must one taste death to know such incredible joy?

August flowed into September, a difficult month emotionally for David as all his friends returned to college, while he couldn't. Weekly visits to the University Hospital in Madison continued. David's hair began to grow back in, and was now curly from his internal chemical permanent.

To fill the void in David's life we began to plan a trip to California to visit Dan Travanti on the Hill Street Blues set. We'd include a visit to family and friends around Los Angeles. The days passed in anticipation.

Finally in November, David reached six months post-transplant and had good blood counts. His cast of eleven months was removed only days before our scheduled departure. Glory of glories, his leg had healed and he could walk without crutches, although he had a limp. It was recommended David use a cane for balance until he became accustomed to walking on two legs again.

David was hugely disappointed. He so wanted to look normal and be normal. How do you tell a young man to walk with the stick of age? We bought a weird, fancy cane and tried to make it fun.

In California we had two days to wait until Dan Travanti would be shooting his scenes on the Hill Street set. The afternoon after our plane arrived Wayne, David, Dan and I glided into the heart of California's Disneyland on a monorail over smooth metallic track. It was a sacred time, like we traveled side by side with God. I felt as if could soar without a transport vehicle.

"Is this really happening?" I exclaimed studying the terrain below. "Thank you Jesus."

Wayne squeezed my hand. "Life doesn't get better than this."

Our fourteen-year-old son Dan beamed. We were thrilled he could enjoy this fun time. Dan had transitioned from seventh to eighth grade during David's illness and made many sacrifices of the lack of our presence, not to mention the hundred of hours he'd spent in hospital visits with his brother.

On the second day on our way back from Disneyland heading to our hotel David said, "Mom, I'm not feeling well."

My body froze. "What's wrong?" David entered the motel room and flopped on the double bed closest to the door. "I'm sick!" Within minutes he was in the washroom vomiting.

David crawled into bed and I took his temperature. He had a low-grade fever.

"Maybe you're just exhausted from all this activity," Wayne said.

"Yeah," David mumbled despondently.

Dr. Longo's instructions regarding any infection were specific. David had to be watched closely, and he was to be called immediately if David's temperature exceeded 101 degrees.

Since transplant whenever David had developed a fever, he'd ended up back in the hospital on antibiotics. I pushed that thought away and struggled to remain calm because I knew a fever accompanied with vomiting was serious.

"David, we can only wait this out, and see what happens. In the meantime, let's make you as comfortable as possible." I plumped his pillow. David's face in repose was frighteningly pale.

We canceled our plans for the evening and turned on the 'IV. Our precious son, Dan, didn't complain at the sudden change. Each of us understood even this minor illness could kill David.

I whispered to Wayne, "How could I have been so foolish as to have thought it safe to come here."

"God's in control in California just as He is in Wisconsin. We need to trust Him," Wayne answered swiftly, but I could tell he was nervous, too.

I called Carla, Dan Travanti's helpful personal secretary, to tell her we couldn't make it the next day. I knew Carla only from our phone contacts as a sweet-voiced woman who exuded efficiency and kindness.

"Carla, David's ill. We'll have to cancel our appointment for tomorrow unfortunately. In fact, I'll need to get him to a hospital tonight if he doesn't improve. Wayne's checking the yellow pages now. We can't go to just any hospital. The staff has to be expert in infectious disease control to treat infection in a patient without an effective immune system."

Carla said, "UCLA has one of the foremost cancer treatment centers in the country. You're about ten minutes away. That's the best place to take your son."

I scribbled down the directions as Carla continued, "I know because I have cancer, too."

I tightened my gripped on the phone to keep from dropping it.

"I'm being treated on an experimental protocol developed at UCLA. The type of cancer I have is very rare. Here's the name of my doctor to use as a reference to expedite getting care for David."

I was incredulous. "Carla, I'm so sorry, I didn't know. You didn't tell me ... "

"I don't discuss my illness often." I heard sadness despite her effort to keep her voice casual.

"How are you doing?"

"So far my protocol is successful, but I have a ways to go."

"Great, Carla, we'll keep you in our prayers. We believe prayer really helps."

"Thanks," Carla said quietly.

"Thank you, Carla. Because of you, the fear of being in an unknown place without an emergency plan has faded."

"Good luck tonight," she said before hanging up.

Wayne and I waited up anxiously, watching and praying till one a.m. This had to be Satan attacking again with both barrels, blasting us with confusion and fear.

We finally went to bed with the alarm set every hour to check David's temperature.

David slept fitfully. Toward morning his fever had left, although he was weak.

"David, your newly developing immune system turned a fever back for the first time without the help of antibiotics!" I said, jumping up exuberantly. "This was to be our day on the Hill Street Blues set. Do you feel up to it?"

We discussed the pros and cons of going and then decided why not. This was initially why we'd come. If necessary, we'd cut short our visit.

David was weak, but enthusiastic.

"Okay, I'll make the arrangements to go to the TV stage."

And what a day we had. We felt like celebrities because we were welcomed so warmly not just by Dan Travanti, but all the cast. Later we had lunch together and spent time visiting at length with Dan in his trailer.

The teeter-totter of illness-health, life-death dropped us with a gentle thud into the comfortable, normal world again.

Mid-January David eagerly returned to the University of Wisconsin-Whitewater. He soon added a new element of excitement to his life and started dating Kathy, a lovely young woman he met in Delavan.

Life was almost like one hopes it can be, but the battle wasn't over yet. A year passed. You'd think that would have been enough time to put this trauma behind, but a new enemy approached from an unforeseen quarter, almost a year to date after transplant.

In the spring of 1987, David lived at a UW-Whitewater college dormitory about forty-five minutes from home as a twenty-year-old freshman. One weeknight after he drove home for dinner, we noticed he was unusually quiet. Wayne asked, "Is something wrong?"

"Mom and Dad, I don't know what's going on with me. I feel incredibly sad, like I want to cry all the time." We tried to lift his spirits but had only moderate success.

David began to come back home from college more often. One minute he'd be fine and the next he was sobbing inconsolably saying things like, "Maybe it would have been better if I'd died during the transplant." Soon he was sleeping at home and commuting to classes.

Over the next week I spent hours counseling David. I'd get him feeling cheerful and positive, but fifteen minutes later, he'd be weeping. I gave him extra Vitamin C to replace the C he was losing from stress. We encouraged him to be outdoors as much as possible, because God uses His natural creation to nurture emotional health. A competent local pastor who did family counseling visited with David also.

Recognizing the signs of clinical depression, I called Dr. Longo. Any treatment or medication David received had to be coordinated through him as primary, follow-up oncologist.

"Doctor, I'm very concerned. As you know, I'm a counselor by profession. My assessment is that David's severely depressed. He's functioning, but barely." I requested an anti-depressant short term.

To my surprise, Dr. Longo replied, "As upsetting as this is, it's not uncommon. We even have a name for it: post-transplant trauma - the depression that comes from surviving transplant. It usually appears one to two years later when a patient dares to believe he's made it through safely."

I listened carefully; surprised such a condition occurred way after the successful medical experience of transplant. Before or during, yes, but up to two years later?

The doctor continued, "The patient's feeling of victory is diminished by the realization of the many losses he's suffered and his practical concerns for the future. Treatment and the passage of time usually alleviates this depression."

We discussed the importance of psychiatric consultation from a Christian perspective, rather than the secular framework at the University Clinic. In the past when I needed to refer clients I recommended Minrith-Meier Clinic in Wheaton, Illinois, despite the distance. I called there and set up an appointment for the following Monday for David to have an evaluation.

Again I called friends for prayers. Faithfully, they responded.

As I put down the phone, I gazed at the placid lake out-side our window. Tremendous activity churned beneath the surface.

I knew that depression was often the outer sign of unacknowledged anger that lingered beneath the surface. After meditating for some time, I wrote David a letter.

"Dear Son,

"I can understand the frustration you must feel. Where are your stolen years of manhood? How can you redeem the weeks of laying your baldhead upon hospital pillows? You can count your losses as others count sheep."

"Where do you find the self-confidence that you lost? Who can lift this stigma of being forever different? These emotional scars are as permanent as the purple radiation markings and the scars upon your body."

"You have a new, young girlfriend in your life. You dare to hope again that there could be long-term happiness, but part of you holds back because you fear another loss, if this relationship becomes too important and is broken."

"What you have already endured reaches out its tentacles to ensnare your restored life. Sparks of ignited fury have no outlet. Who can be blamed? Where do you put the unspoken anger that you had to submit to the indignity of treatment, anger at the doctors and nurses who healed you, yet inflicted pain, anger at a greedy economic structure in our country that polluted your environment, anger at God who allowed you to suffer. Anger at employers, who won't hire you because of your medical history?"

"School isn't the same. You're too old to fit in with freshman; the older students know you've matured beyond them and you do, too. You can't go back to what you missed in the normal sequence of life."

"Yes, son, I understand. New emotional conflicts rip apart your efforts at emotional equanimity. You've gone now from taking one day at a time to planning for a lifetime."

"For this, too, God gives grace, but first we must face the problem."

Writing helped me see the magnitude of these negative feelings we'd never discussed together. I never sent the letter.

The next Monday I drove David two and one half hours to Minrith-Meier Clinic. When we walked in we discovered the schedule had gone awry because of the attempted suicide of a client seen just prior to David's appointment.

After an hour wait in a packed reception room, David was finally called back. Less than forty-five minutes later, a female Indian psychiatrist in her forties, approached me.

"I've given David a thorough evaluation. It's my opinion that he does not need hospitalization. However, outpatient group work for depression would be beneficial. He needs to work through unfinished grief over his experiences of the last two years - feel it, taste it, and then let go."

I nodded.

She continued, "I've recommended several books on grieving that I think will help. Call me in two weeks," the psychiatrist concluded.

Out in the fresh air again, I breathed deeply, waiting for David's response. He was deep in thought.

Finally I asked, "David would you like to come back here for group therapy?"

"No, that's not necessary, Mom. I can work through my grief with you. I realize now I haven't done that completely. I know God will have the final victory, but I've been trying to ignore losses that can't be ignored."

All the long drive home, David and I took turns reciting a litany of our feelings during each horrible thing that had happened over the past two years. We hadn't focused on the emotional trauma before; we were too busy coping. During the transplant a positive focus was necessary, but now it was time to touch the pain. In my mind I added a P.S. to my letter. "Where is the punching bag that can absorb your fury? Grieve my son, weep, and we will weep with you." I described for the first time Wayne's pain and mine as well. We relived all the most horrible incidents. David cried, I cried. At times I could barely see the road through flooded eyes.

Within days David was back to his joyful self. He's never again been troubled with such deep torment.

Now with heart-stopping awe I watch David work, study, laugh, run. And I remember the words quoted by my son-in-law that I'd struggled against at the start of these perilous days. "Whatsoever you ask for in prayer, believe that ye may receive."

What does this mean if not that we are to trust in God rather than in evidence of what we see?

And then I remember Wayne's persistent pleas to God.

"Faith is the assurance of things hoped for–ASSURANCE." (Hebrews 11:1) "Yet shall he live!"

Thank you, Jesus. We have seen a miracle.

TIMELINE

1986 – David is told by two oncologists he has less than 24 hours to live.

1987 - 1991 – David returns to college and graduates with honors from University of Wisconsin.

1992 – David marries Kathleen Kane.

1992 - 1994 – David attends Graduate School, Virginia Beach, VA and is selected as Most Outstanding Public Policy Graduate.

1995 - 2000 – David completes doctoral studies in History at Florida State University and becomes a history teacher.

2004 – David and his wife Kathy become the parents of twins, Anna and Joshua Rolfs.

2011 – David writes acclaimed book on spirituality and the Civil War called *No Peace for the Wicked,* published by University of Tennessee Press.

EPILOGUE

People have asked if David was healed by prayer or by modern medicine. My answer is both.

Was it a miracle? Yes.

Is prayer effective? You must decide what you believe based on what you have read.

Some have thought that David simply got lucky. Twice he was pronounced within hours of death, once twenty-four and then four hours. Both these times, the coincidental circumstances through which his life was saved were too numerous and unusual to attribute God's spectacular intervention to mere chance.

We don't discount the magnificent dedication and expertise of the attending doctors. But even they warned against giving them all the credit. They can perform identical procedures on two different patients with vastly different results. Many doctors acknowledge the operation of a Power outside their control that makes the life or death difference for patients.

If you are going through this battle you'll need to use every tool God has given for the fight. Your own intelligence, intuition, and fortitude are essential. Dig deep for the best information you can gather.

Pray for wisdom, minute by minute, in every decision.

Pray before, during and after treatments. Ask your community of believers to pray. Search Scripture and use every principle that applies from the Gospel message of healing. The principles work, because they are God's order for man. Do your homework. The stance of Christ on healing is not hidden. The words of Jesus are true. He's the Supreme Healer. It takes more energy to alter His words than to apply them as truth. Time after time, Jesus healed out of compassion, not merely to show His power as God. He often told those He healed to go and tell no one. Yet, He knew His miracles attracted multitudes to His message of eternal life - the most important gift he offers. Temporal healing of the physical body is a minor act compared to the wondrous growth of a relationship with Jesus leading to eternal life.

"Seek ye first the kingdom of heaven and its righteousness, and all other things will be added unto you." (Matthew 6:33) To be in the Kingdom of heaven is to be in the presence of God and to know Him.

Ask for healing. God's Word says, "Until now you have asked nothing in My name; ask, and you will receive, that your joy may be full." (John 16:24) and "Pray without ceasing." (1Thessalonians 5: 17) and "Whatever things you ask in prayer, believing, you will receive." (Matthew 21: 22)

Jesus said not to worry, not to fear, but to live in joy long before Norman Vincent Peale spoke of the power of positive thinking. Jesus suggested we eliminate guilt and bitterness from our lives before psychologists talked about the power that exists within the mind.

Some promote using a spirit guide, calling on angels, dabbling in ungodly spirits. But you need to be careful you don't mix your spirits. Almighty God does not share godhead with other gods, angels or man. He may send a ministering angel, but you can't summon one.

The one thing Jesus always requested of His followers was belief and trust in Him. God responds to faith. Noah, Abraham, David, Daniel, all had to trust totally in God to do the impossible, which He did time and again. God insisted on belief before the results were manifested in their lives.

How much faith is enough? Jesus said very little. As parents we weren't totally free of fear and worry when David was ill. It took an ongoing act of our will to control anxiety and not be controlled by it, when we waited for doctor's reports. Like a rubber ball, temptation toward disbelief kept bouncing back.

Where do you get faith in the first place? Faith comes from hearing the Word of God, and acting on the Word of God. It helps to remember little moments of God's faithfulness in the past and blend them with trust for the future. Faith is not something you develop and carry around in a shopping bag for life. Like the sun's rays, it must be new each day. When you need more, it's highly contagious from the faith of others. Guilt, bitterness and fear make faith cringe and wither.

Prayer deepens faith. Answered prayer increases it.

Have you ever wondered, how long should you pray? How many prayers does it take for a miracle?

We don't know. That's up to God. We have learned, that if the results have not yet appeared, it obviously takes more. Intercessory prayer may be the most powerful and neglected ministry within the church.

Pray continuously.

Job lost his family, then his possessions, finally his health. Yet he never lost his faith in God. You can't be wishy-washy pray-ers. God always hears and always answers one way or another. His solutions are put into motion instantly, but we must wait for their enactment in time. He may not always do as you wish.

David became worse, before he got better. As egocentric humans we wanted our way immediately. Instead we learned to trust God's way wherever He led. When we relinquish all to Him, we receive what's best for our lives.

"Why is there physical and emotional sickness?" My counseling clients have often asked me this question. "For the same reasons that sin happens," I answer. "The sources of both are the world, the flesh, and the devil."

Yes, Satan fires off his best shots to knock out the faith of God's people. Well, Satan, go back to hell. God pulled us through the mire, and even made it good.

Romans 8:28 is a verse of truth upon which you can stake your life. "We know that all things work for good for those who love God, who are called according to His purpose." I believe we are better parents, better mates, and I hope better friends to others because of our increased sensitivity to others' pain as a result of our own.

Praise God, not for the pain, nor for the horror of suffering and sickness, but because, no matter what, He alone can and does make good come from all things, even evil. "His banner over us is love." (Song of Solomon 2:4) You, too, will see the good come.

Why are some not healed? I don't know. Sometimes a loved one dies suddenly before you have time to pray or study the word on healing. Only God knows why death comes so quickly. Other times there is a long, lingering illness. In every situation God is sovereign. For a believer, whenever death comes, eternal life with God is the delightful reward.

I know it's easier to be faith-filled when you're not in constant pain. That's why the Body of Christ, the community, is so important. Read about the paralyzed man whose friends brought him to Jesus by lowering him through the roof. Jesus said because of their faith he would heal the man. When a person is sick they often lack the positive resources to practice faith. Their energy is consumed in coping day by day.

The faith and prayers of the community of family and friends strengthen the faith of the sick person and add to his confidence and spiritual strength. They convey God's healing and hope. Jesus said, "Greater works than those I have done you will do, when the

Holy Spirit comes upon you." That's through His power, not the power of humans.

Some people truly don't seek healing. I've never been surprised at Jesus' question to the sick, "What do you want?" or the Scripture that reads, "You have not, because you ask not."

There are times when the consequences of infirmity can be more rewarding particularly to a member of a dysfunctional family. Extra attention, sympathy, release from responsibilities, having demands met without argument can be attractive tradeoffs. Sometimes, a patient needs counseling to become aware of these deeper motives for embracing sickness. God does not intrude with healing in such lives.

Some, not all, sickness comes from people's sins. Jesus told the man to get up and walk; his sins were forgiven. Forgiveness is readily available.

In our minds we went back through David's life stage by stage, and asked forgiveness for his sins, and for parenting errors and sins of my husband and myself. We prayed that God heal the whole of David, body, mind, and soul and He did.

Some are not healed because they simply lack knowledge of the healing activity of God. "You have not because you ask not."

What's required is total submission to the mystery of God. The Almighty, omnipotent God will allow and do whatever He pleases.

While healing may not always happen, it should happen far more than it does. It is usually God's perfect plan for man, but free will being totally free, man can abuse self and others. For example, David could have been killed instantly in the car accident. We've learned, too, to pray daily for God's protection on our loved ones.

Sometimes, quite simply, healing doesn't happen because there comes a time when your purpose in life is completed. All people eventually die. Perhaps God has decided a person has achieved the ultimate level of development in his earthly relationships, and now he shall see His face. When do you quit asking? When Jesus impresses upon you and your loved ones it's time to move on without bitterness or anxiety.

God chose to take our eighteen-year-old son, David, from the cross of cancer, and restore his life. David went to God in trust and submitted. Jesus became the Word made flesh crucified for our sins and our sicknesses and ultimately gave the Word, that is, "Say but the Word and he shall be healed."

All his life, David will remember that Jesus saved him and that Jesus loves him. In some way, which we don't yet know, David's life will be different and radiant because he carries the healing touch of God.

David does not look back. But his mind and soul have been branded with God's mark, so that honoring God is David's foremost desire. He has won acclaim from philosophy and history professors for his excellent research against abortion and evolution. David is God's man, now and forever a defender of God's Word and Christian truth. His career is in history and public policy.

We thank God for the privilege of witnessing a miracle.

In awe, we remember the prophetic words spoken about our son, David, by a godly man in prayer, "Yet shall he live."

We want to tell the world so that they too have reason for hope. We're committed to proclaiming the controversial truth - God is God of the impossible. Nothing is too difficult for him.

But, the most important question for you today is the same one Jesus asked Peter. "Whom do you say that I am?" Lord? Savior? Bearer of our sins and our sicknesses? What do you choose to believe? Will it be the Word spoken by God, or the fabrications made by man based on their own lack of faith or unwillingness to pray faithfully? If His words are true, God alone is exalted, not man.

Who do you say Jesus is? Miracle working Son of God or an audacious has-been from another age with an unpleasant message about death to self and finding a fuller life through Him. If you haven't fully surrendered your life to Christ perhaps now is the time to make Him your Lord and Savior.

As for us, we will tell the world, not just that Jesus healed our son, but that everyone can seek healing and trust the results to God's perfect will. We inhale deeply and proclaim the controversial message that Jesus Christ is the same yesterday, today, and forever. He is the truth and He spoke the truth when He said, "Greater works than these, you shall do when I leave." (John 14:12) Not for just a decade or a century, but always.

To God be the glory, David lives.

Triumphing Over Cancer:

Patient & Caregiver's Forty Survival Strategies

These strategies may seem somewhat radical. Yet the methods described are totally accepted in the medical and spiritual communities.

I researched healing extensively when our eighteen-year-old son David was stricken with T-cell leukemia and became one of the first successful bone marrow transplant patients. My studies in Psychology and Marriage and Family Counseling along with a lifelong fascination with the workings of the human body all came into consideration.

I became intrigued by how the healing process is influenced on two levels – the physical and the spiritual. Psychoneuroimmunology, a long medical term, is the respected study of the interaction between psychological processes and the nervous and immune systems of the human body. Quite simply what you feel, think and believe can and does influence your ability to fight disease. This is proven fact.

Visualization, that is seeing things in your mind before they exist in reality, is powerful. Scripture refers to this phenomenon in the Gospel of Mark Chapter 11: Verse 24. "Whatsoever you ask for in prayer, believe that you will receive it."

I also studied the amazing healing miracles of Jesus. Many times Jesus Christ referred to the faith of the individual as powerful in their healing. "Go your way. Your faith has saved you." (Gospel of Luke

150

Chapter 7, verse 50) The reality of the power of prayer, enlisting the action of God the Father, Son and Holy Spirit is a huge factor in the healing process. I'm not saying prayer is hocus-pocus words, not at all, it's connecting your mind and heart to God's.

In a nutshell, I prayed and believed for God's healing power to be released. I also encouraged my son to visualize every drip of the chemo entering his body as destroying only cancer cells while not impacting one single healthy cell. I prayed privately and with others repeatedly for the healing of our son. Prayer was a privilege and gave me an active role in what might have otherwise been a depressing, helpless vigil. Doctors later confirmed they had thought our son's illness was hopeless and admitted that they witnessed an amazing occurrence of healing.

God's will is sovereign, His will may be to show His power and demonstrate His love in a palpable way by healing you or your loved one. Or God may have determined your life purpose or your loved one's has been completed now. We all must die of something, some day, but let it not be one day before we are meant to.

God often uses illness and suffering to open the minds and hearts of patients or caregivers or others in their immediate surroundings who have been hardened to His love, or who have become indifferent or denied His existence.

These strategies can accompany you during your own journey. Never stop seeking healing. On the contrary, fight illness with every bit of your strength, hence the title *Triumphing Over Cancer*. I pray healing will be yours for body as well as your soul.

Forty Survival Strategies

1. When You First Hear the News
2. When You Wonder Why
3. When You're Scared
4. When You Want To Withdraw
5. When You're Discouraged
6. When You're Confused About Medical Options
7. When You Need More Joy
8. When Treatment Makes You Ill
9. When Things Go Wrong
10. When You Lack Confidence In Your Doctor
11. When You Need A Boost
12. When You Need To Relax
13. When You Feel Like A Number
14. When "If -Onlys" Attack
15. When You're In Pain
16. When You're Grumpy
17. When You Feel Forgotten
18. When You're Bored
19. When You Need Cheering
20. When You Feel Family Tension
21. When You Need More Support
22. When You Need Assurance
23. When You Miss the Familiar
24. When You Need Some Fun
25. When You're Tired
26. When You Need Inspiration
27. When You Want To Be A Giver
28. When You're Bitter
29. When You Overdo
30. When Your Schedule Is Overwhelming
31. When You Wonder If God Can Help
32. When You Feel Down
33. When You Question God
34. When You Feel Guilty

Appendix

1. When You First Hear the News

The first days are almost unendurable. You want to slip into unreality and pretend that nothing's happened, that the diagnosis isn't true.

But it is. And panic strikes. What do you do first? A million thoughts flood your mind.

Start with God. Reassure yourself that God knows and God cares. Accept His comfort as you pray for strength and restored health.

Request His wisdom as you make choices pursuing the best treatment.

"I will cry unto God Most High, unto God that performeth aft things for me. Me shaft send from heaven and save me... God shaft send forth His mercy and His truth." Ps. 57:2-3 (KJV)

2. When You Wonder Why

One of the first things you'll face is getting past the "Whys." Why did you get this terrible disease? What went wrong? Was it poor diet, exposure to a cancer-causing chemical, too much stress, too little exercise?

Chances are there is not a direct tie-in between something you did or didn't do and this illness. If there's a link as in the case of smoking and lung cancer, what happened in the past is done. Accept that and move on. You can't waste energy on self - recrimination. Since God forgives your mistakes, you can forgive yourself, too.

Why you anyway? Are you too nice, too easy-going? Should you have expressed your feelings more strongly? Learned how to deal with stress better? That's what some psychotherapists might say. Should you have been more spiritual? That's what some ministers might say – similar to the comfort Job received from his friends - useless speculation and painful condemnation.

Who knows? There are no definitive answers. You could struggle endlessly with these questions. You aren't perfect, but you're in the process of becoming more Christ-like. That's all God asks of you.

The best advice is talk through these feelings with your caregiver, then forget about the "whys" and focus on the "hows" of healing. "Cheer up. Take courage if you're depending on the Lord." (Psalm 31:24 NKJV)

3. When You're Scared

It's natural to be afraid. Can you get through treatment? What side effects will there be? Can you do nothing and chance living without treatment?

Over and over Scripture reminds you not to harbor fear. Excessive fear wastes your precious energy; fear can't help you. People conquer cancer every day, and you can be among them! Refuse thoughts of death or permanent disability.

Use your energy instead to explore all your treatment options with the help of your caregiver if you have one. If you don't, ask God to send someone to support you through this. You may be surprised at who the Lord brings to the forefront of your life.

May you be encouraged by this verse from Scripture: "God is our [my] refuge and strength, an ever present help in trouble. 'Therefore we [I] will not fear, though the earth give way and the mountains fall into the heart of the sea, though its waters roar and foam and the mountains quake with their surging." (Psalm 46: 9 NKJV)

4. When You Want to Withdraw

Use every resource God has given, your own intelligence, intuition, and fortitude are essential. Dig deep for every weapon - the best information, medically and spiritually. Let not the Master find that you have slacked off, and left all your work to Him. Do your part and He'll do His. Healing comes from prayer, positive mental attitude, and modem medicine.

If you're able to, memorize Psalm 103. You'll find great comfort there. Perhaps your <u>caregiver</u> can get it copied in large type on 81/2 by 11 paper that you can hold while you memorize it and post it in your room.

5. When You're Discouraged

You can't control the physical surroundings of being in a hospital or clinic, but you can transform your mental surroundings by the thoughts you think. Wherever you are, whatever's happening, you can have more influence on your surroundings than they have on you.

Think future when the present seems unbearable. Fill your mind with facts about other individual's experiences of healing.

Think about the kindness of the people around you. Perhaps your caregiver can collect some resources summarizing the stories of other patients who have been healed of cancer.

"Whatsoever is good, pure and true, these things you shall think about." (Philippians 4:8 9, KJV)

6. When You're Confused About Medical Options

You can have a powerful voice in your care. Don't be intimidated by a lack of prior knowledge about cancer. Get the information you need to co-operate in decision-making and make informed choices from the facts available. Doctors, themselves, admit they often don't know what is absolutely best. Even they must make educated guesses.

If you get stressed when discussing your illness with doctors, bring a tape recorder to record their diagnosis and treatment plan.

Until you genuinely understand a procedure, ask for as many explanations as required from your own doctor, other staff doctors, nurses, and technicians. You need to know all your options.

Once you understand and agree to a treatment, co-operate with it whole-heartedy physically, emotionally, and spiritually. Your caregiver can help. Different clinics often recommend different protocols depending on the research specializations of their staff. If you're feeling too ill to research these, ask family members or friends to gather additional information for you. They can call cancer hotlines and contact the major cancer centers for their latest approaches.

Ask your family members to participate in medical conferences concerning your care so that they can help you understand and remember the recommendations made. Use a tape recorder if necessary. "Blessed is the man who finds wisdom, the man who gains understanding... She is a tree of life to those who embrace her; those who lay hold of her will be blessed." (Proverbs 3:13,18)

7. When You Need More Joy

You can focus your attitude in any direction you choose. There is documented evidence that positive attitude and good feelings actually trigger increased immunoglobulins, which are an essential part of the body's defense and rehabilitation systems. In medical terms this is called psychoneuroimmunology. It's real and it works.

Choose to foster a positive attitude and good feelings to facilitate your recovery. Try to bless another person in some specific way. Through an affirming word, humorous comment, heartfelt prayer, you, too, can give help to others even as you receive help.

Recognize the importance of prayer and effectively use your quiet times to pray for yourself and the needs of others. These may be patients, doctors, nurses, your caregiver, other patients if you're hospitalized or family and friends.

The very fact that you're reading this book is evidence that you're pursuing a positive spirit and every aspect leading toward healing. Excellent!

Over and over test the amazing, mysterious, and truthful Scripture assurance: "And we know that all things work together for good to those who love God, to those who are the called according to His purpose. (Romans 8:28, NIV)

8. When Treatment Makes You Ill

When you're feeling very weary or sick remember that it's seldom the cancer that has created this feeling; more often it's the powerful methods that are used to push cancer away. Visualize the drugs and procedures working powerfully to eradicate the cancer. Remind yourself that these physical feelings of illness are temporary and ultimately beneficial.

With God's grace you can endure. It helps to have your caregiver reassure you at these times.

All things will pass.

"I can do all things through Christ who strengthens me." (Phil. 4:13 NKJV)

9. When Things Go Wrong

After agreeing with a plan of care or treatment, continue to seek information as to its progress. If the initial outcomes are not as you anticipated or unresolvable complications occur, evaluate and choose appropriate alternatives.

Even if you're part of a study group used to research a type of treatment, drop out if something more positive appears. Studies often have missing cases. Don't hesitate to change your mind if it's in you best interest. Ask your caregiver to be present for moral support whenever you need to confront your doctors about current treatment procedures. At times your caregiver may even need to do the talking for you.

Pray for wisdom in making decisions. Then depend upon the fact that "He that is perfect in knowledge is with thee." (Job 36:4)

10. When You Lack Confidence In Your Doctor

Let your doctor know your emotional concerns and personal needs. Keep an honest, open relationship with him or her. If your doctor doesn't inspire your hope and encourage your own positive approach toward healing, find another doctor. Hope is immeasurably important.

If you don't believe that you have the best doctor for your type of cancer or that you will receive the best possible physical and emotional treatment, find another doctor.

If your form of cancer has not historically responded well to standard, established protocol, have friends or family call other major cancer centers for information. Your caregiver can see what types of experimental protocols are available. Don't hesitate to participate in any reasonable alternative treatment that appears promising.

"But if the Spirit of Him who raised Jesus from the dead dwells in you, He who raised Christ from the dead will also give life to your mortal bodies through His Spirit who dwells in you." (Romans 8:11)

11. When You Need A Boost

Visualize yourself as healthy. This is simply controlled daydreaming. Imagine yourself in a moving picture frame of life involved in the different activities you enjoy: conversing with dear ones; dining out at your favorite restaurant; running along the ocean; sitting on the verandah of a hotel.

In all these pictures, perceive yourself as fully present. See your body as strong and supple. Tell yourself you'll be that way again.

If you need help to imagine these scenes, ask your caregiver to bring snapshots, travel brochures, or magazine pictures to help you form mental pictures with yourself as the star.

"If we hope for what we do not see, we eagerly wait for it with perseverance." (Romans 8:25)

12. When You Need To Relax

Your relaxation is essential. Engage in some physical activity each day. Even if you're confined to bed, you can concentrate upon contracting and releasing your muscles. Enjoy the sensations of your body as muscles are stretched.

If you're up to it, walk outdoors. Walking is the perfect exercise because you can adjust it to any level of exertion that is right for you.

Remember that laughter is excellent exercise. Ask your caregiver to rent funny movies, arrange for you to listen to comedian's tapes, radio shows and read cartoon books. Surround yourself with people who will share your fun.

Learn daily the sublime lesson of trust and calm in the midst of storm.

"Whatever of sorrow or difficulty the day may bring, my tender command to you is still the same – love and laugh." from <u>GOD CALLING</u> July 1st written by Two Listeners, edited by A. J. Russell, Barbour Books.

13. When You Feel Like A Number

Consider your unique needs during the course of medical treatment. Occasionally you'll need to be an exception to hospital meal or rest schedules for your physical comfort or emotional nurture. Strongly request that you be accommodated. With fondness and firmness, you can control some of these aspects of your life. Be good to yourself.

If you're feeling depressed or totally out of control, don't hesitate to express it. Request the physical and emotional support you need. There are times in everyone's life when they must accept being dependent upon others. Don't play the games of pride or false humility. Request and accept help from your faithful caregiver and other family members and friends with gratitude.

You may not be able to choose all that happens to you these days; but you can control some events and how you react to them.

"When pride comes, then comes shame; but with the humble is wisdom." (Proverbs **11**:**2**)

14. When The "If-Onlys" Attack

Each new day means more hours to pass. Many things may be out of your control, but not <u>every</u> thing. Refuse the tempting, dangerous contemplation of the "if only's." Be determined to think and act as if you expect blessings and restored health.

Fear, anger and sadness are sweetly beckoning but dangerous demons. Don't let them in.

Look for gladness; it's there somewhere if you dig deeply. Search for and savor glimmers of joy in your moment-by-moment experiences. Meditate on verses like Romans 8:28 "All things work together for good for those who love the Lord and are called according to His purpose."

15. When You're In Pain

If you must endure pain or other discomfort that can't be completely controlled by medication, find a rhythm and harmony to it. View it as a positive signal from a healing body alerting all inner physical, emotional, and spiritual forces to restorative action.

Pain is...a mountain peak to scale.

Pain is...a wild stallion you ride.

Pain is... how would you describe it? Write your answer.

Remember always:

Pain is...temporary.

Meditate on these encouraging verses from the Message Bible: "I'm hurt and in pain. Give me space for healing and mountain air. Let me shout God's name with a praising song. Let me tell his greatness in a prayer of thanks." Psalm 69:29-36

16. When You're Grumpy

Make an effort to see something beautiful today and every day. You may have to work at it, but do it! Then share what you find with someone who visits or write a letter if you're all alone.

Sharing an experience of beauty with someone else enriches you, too, in some mysterious way. Talk freely about what you appreciate; dwell on whatever is beautiful in people and in your surroundings.

"The happiness of life is made up of minute fractions - the little, soon-forgotten charities of a kiss, a smile, a kind look, a heartfelt compliment in the disguise of a playful raillery, and the countless other infinitesimals of pleasant thought and feeling." Samuel Taylor Coleridge

17. When You're Afraid God Has Forgotten You

God never does forget you, you know. Try to remember treasured places and experiences where you've felt a sense of the awe of God. Maybe it's a favorite woodland of virgin white birch trees on a velvet table of grass; match sticks of moonlight like candlelight; flames of sunlight piercing dusty shadows; memories of wind tickling your ears.

Reflect on these moments of knowing unmistakable union with our majestic creative God.

Nature is a great reminder of God's presence in the world.

"He has made everything beautiful in its time."
(Ecclesiastes 3:11)

18. When You're Bored

Everyone possesses creative gifts of some kind. Try releasing your creative force even if you've never considered yourself creative before. Write a story about an interesting or humorous anecdote. Make tapes of your conversations with medical staff, and add silly, humorous comments later. Your visitors will appreciate them.

Try needlework or paint portraits or draw cartoons - yes, even if you've never drawn before. Maybe you'd enjoy putting together birdhouses or clock kits.

There are interesting ways to pass this time of limited activity that can bring you creative satisfaction. Don't stop experimenting until you find some creative outlet you enjoy.

This is a great time to develop new skills and interests; you may discover gifts during these days that will enrich your future life.

Our creative God made us in His image and likeness with His creative abilities as recorded in Genesis.

19. When You Need Cheering

Welcome joy, humor and lightheartedness. You can set the tone of your environment. - humorous stories, booths, video movies - can lighten your heart. Let your caregiver and other loved ones know you want your home or hospital room to be a cheery, not somber, place.

Invite friends who bring cheerful, uplifting conversation.

Visitors who bring something to smile or laugh about bring friends' gifts greater than frankincense, gold, and myrrh or any gift money can buy. Your family's assistance will be helpful in selecting booths, magazines, travel brochures, etc. for you and your guests to enjoy.

Kindly discourage visits from friends or family members who depress you. Choose your companions carefully.

"Happiness is reflective of the light of heaven." Washington Irving.

20. When You Feel Family Tension

A time of illness is an excellent time to strengthen or restore, if necessary, important personal relationships in your life. Calls, notes, or visits can express your gratitude to the family members and friends, whose unique qualities have added to your life. Resolve any tensions that may have existed by honest sharing of past hurts followed by a willingness to forgive. Ask for your caregiver's assistance with this.

Examine your past life year by year, and ask God to take away any sin from you. Sweep away any lingering specks of bitterness or resentment - every form - any trace. It can weight your body immeasurably and prevent your flight to freedom from disease. Reject bitterness as the plague!

"Pursue peace with all people, and holiness, Without which no one will see the Lord: looking carefully lest anyone fall short of the grace of God; lest any root of bitterness springing up cause trouble, and by this many become defiled." (Hebrews 12:14-15)

21. When You Need More Family Support

Unfortunately family members sometimes prepare themselves prematurely for a loved one's death as a sort of psychological protection. Ask your family to act as partners in your fight for life, instead of wasting their energy and yours, by contemplating your loss to them.

If necessary, have your caregiver or medical staff personnel inform your family that they're acting selfishly and harmfully by preparing to mourn instead of preparing to celebrate life with you.

Ask your caregiver and other loved ones to pray daily without ceasing for your total recovery.

"Rejoice always. Pray without ceasing." (1 Thess. 5:16-17)

22. When You Need Assurance

I hope and pray every person who reads *Triumphing Over Cancer* will experience God's tender, loving touch. You'll draw infinitely closer to Him as you study His ways and feel His assurance. One thing is true, whatever happens, God loves you! I'll say it again, He loves you! When you turn the controls of your life over to Him, He'll give you only the very best. Believe this and trust no matter what. May you have a long and joyful life, spreading the news wherever you go of our wondrous Father God's healing mercy and love.

At various times during your treatment, you'll need human reassurance also. You may be more down and less physically active. You'll be even more sensitive to the words you hear in your private world. Be discriminating regarding the tone, style, and content of these sound symbols and note their effect on you. Think about the wisdom in the following Proverbs and perhaps post them as reminders for your visitors.

"There are those who speak rashly like the piercing of a sword, but the tongue of the wise brings healing." (Proverbs 12:18)

"Pleasant words are as a honeycomb, sweet to the soul, and health to the bones."(Proverbs 16:24)

23. When You Miss The Familiar

If hospitalization is sometimes necessary during your treatment, ask your family to help you personalize your hospital surroundings no matter how short the stay. Try to create a setting with touches of home. Bring your favorite pillow and most comfortable bedding. Perhaps bring a tape recorder with taped sounds of familiar comfort like the birds outside your kitchen window, the waves from a special lake site, your dog barking.

Have someone check with the hospital staff for their guidelines regarding hanging pictures, humorous posters, bringing silk flowers (real ones are usually not allowed).

Encourage your caregiver or other family members to bring pictures of you in action doing favorite things. Tape them everywhere - even in the bathroom! These reminders of real life will take you beyond the world of institutionalized living that can be so dehumanizing. You need to feel more human and precious than ever before, because you are precious. God desires that you be comforted in every way possible during this difficult time.

"Behold what manner of love the Father has bestowed on us that we should be called children of God!" (1 John 3:1)

24. When You Need More Fun

Fun is essential in life. You can still be a fun person when hospitalized. Don't be afraid to be different. Doing the unexpected occasionally helps brighten your day and reminds staff you're not a case study, but a human being. When our eighteen-year-old son was hospitalized for cancer treatment, a friend brought him a squirt gun. He used it on anyone who entered his hospital room until the head nurse took it away when the floor became too slippery.

Humorous or unusual signs on your door will make medical staff want to enter your room wondering what's going on in there. They create a wonderful, relaxed air. Fun signs might be: "Do not enter these premises have been condemned." "Explosives ahead!" "Closed for vacation. Back next week!" With the focus on fun hospital staff will find visiting your room more pleasant, which in turn may make them more pleasant and accommodating. These fun-filled moments are truly conducive to healing.

If you're too ill to plan fun things, ask your caregiver or other friends to participate in the details of arranging good times.

The discomforting side effects of cancer treatments can usually be controlled medically, thank God. But occasionally depression is an annoying result of some chemotherapy drugs. Light-hearted, shared fun can take your mind off your treatment and brighten your spirit.

"A cheerful heart causeth good healing, but a broken spirit drieth up the bones." (Proverbs 17:22)

25. When You're Tired

Sleep is an amazing restorative process. Sometimes you'll be sedated prior to receiving chemotherapy treatments and you may be extremely exhausted afterwards. In either case, relish these times of extra repose as intense healing periods.

You may find that classical or popular music provides a soothing background for you during and after treatment. Music can be an essential aspect of healing as it was for King Saul when the shepherd, David, played for him, before Saul broke off their relationship. Let music soothe you to sleep.

"When thou liest down, thou shalt not be afraid: yea, thou shalt lie down, and thy sleep shall be sweet." (Proverbs 3:24)

"Thou shalt be secure, because there is hope... and thou shalt take thy rest in safety" (Job 11:18)

26. When You Need Inspiration

If you study God's role in the creation of world and specifically the human body, you'll come to the conclusion that God is the original designer of the complexity and intricacy of life. Since God made it, He has the ability to repair it.

Many reputable Christian and non-Christian scientists admit that God alone holds the secret of life.

To ignore God's role in the restoration of health is foolishness. The Old and New Testament hold the wisdom of the centuries regarding the living conditions that will keep you safe from mental and physical illness. This is the wisdom you need to regain to sustain your health.

God says that his Word (Scripture) and the principles therein can directly affect the length of your life:

"Set your hearts on all the words which I testify among you this day, which you shall command your children to be careful to serve, all the words of this law. For it is no vain thing for you; because it is your life and through this thing, you shall prolong your days." (Deuteronomy 32:46-47)

27. When You Want To Be A Giver

Even if your total savings is $100, you can give 10% or $10 and find two people or charities to benefit from $5. Not every gift has to be huge or tax deductible. Give more if you're able. All money belongs ultimately to God and He's always a generous giver. Scripture talks about the benefits of tithing - giving ten per cent of your earnings to caring for others or the work of the church.

Isaiah 58:7 & 8 suggest the importance of dividing your bread with the hungry, clothing the naked, and to "Hide, not yourself from the needs of your own flesh and blood."

There's a mental release that comes from not clinging too tightly to material blessings. Ultimately nothing monetary will enter eternal life with you. Only the good deeds you've done on behalf of Christ will have any value once you have left earthly life. Build treasures for yourself in heaven where neither moth or rust can destroy.

The anticipated result of these actions is revealed in Isaiah 58, verse 8: "Then shall your light break forth as the morning, and your healing, your restoration and the power of a new life shall spring forth speedily; your rightness, your justice, and your right relationship with God shall go before you conducting you to peace and prosperity, and the glory of the Lord shall be your rearguard."

28. When You're Bitter

The temporary satisfaction that comes from harboring a negative emotion like bitterness isn't worth its destructive effects upon your body.

The Scriptural principles about living in peace and harmony contribute to health, because they are God's order for man. You may need to talk these things through with your caregiver, or a professional counselor if they persist.

It's wise to check the state of your mind and heart daily for these dangerous, negative emotions. Forgive yourself as well as others for any past wrongs. If you refuse to take offense, no one can hurt you emotionally.

Perhaps write a note encouraging someone you scarcely know who has served you in the past - maybe a local business. Call someone you know and tell them something you admire about them.

Although your body may be temporarily incapacitated, your mind and heart are strong and vigorous. Use them today. Be a giver and a taker from the well of life.

"A calm and undisturbed mind and heart are the life and health of the body, but envy, jealousy, and wrath are as rottenness of the bones." (Proverbs 14:30)

29. When You Overdo

Rest times each day need to be a regular procedure in your schedule, not hit or miss depending on other circumstances. And rest means true rest -not a lapful of paperwork or yard work if you're physically able, unless you love those things. Competitive sports and games are great if you feel up to them and they don't drain your energy excessively.

Every day try to get an extra 3-4 hours of rest. That's about one-seventh of your day. And pay attention to your thoughts. Make sure they stay positive.

"Commune with your own heart upon your bed, and be still." (Psalm 4:4)

"Finally, brothers, whatever is true, whatever is noble, whatever is right, whatever is pure, whatever is lovely, whatever is admirable—if anything is excellent or praiseworthy—think about such things." Philippians 4:8 (NIV)

30. When Your Schedule Is Overwhelming

Even during your busiest season at your job and at home, you need rest on the seventh day to maintain your health. Whether it's a Sunday or Saturday Sabbath, whichever you observe, you need a daylong period of rest.

The Sabbath is to be a day of genuine renewal to refresh you from the previous week's activities and energize you for the future. Originally the one and only disciplined activity during the Sabbath was reading and reflecting on the law of God.

Sunday or the Sabbath is to be a designed day as a source of joy. Revel in it with your caregiver and other loved ones.

Scripture says: "Six days you shall work but on the seventh day you shaft rest; even in p lowing time and in harvests, you shaft rest on the seventh day." ('Exodus 34:21)

31. When You Wonder If God Can Help

All of Scripture focuses on God's relationship with His people and their faith response to Him. Faith is the one quality most praised by God, even the smallest iota of trust in God's healing love for you.

To strengthen your faith, read the life story of Hezekiah who was healed from terminal illness through seething God's intervention. He went on to live an additional fifteen years. (2 Kings 20) after experiencing God's healing.

Hopefully you can find at least one Christian friend or family member, ideally your <u>caregiver,</u> and if possible three or four more who will believe with you and for you for God's divine healing.

Matthew 11:24 "Therefore, I say unto you, What things so ever ye desire, when you pray, believe that you receive them, and you shall have them."

32. When You Feel Down

Do you believe you deserve this illness because you're inadequate as a human being? Wrong! Perhaps you believe you've failed in some area of importance to your marriage or a job. This may be true, and it may or may not have been your fault but it isn't the reason you got cancer.

If you're Christian, consider the answer of Jesus to those who asked him what sins of Lazarus had caused his sickness. Jesus said, "This sickness is not a result of Lazarus' sins nor is it unto death, but only that God be glorified through the healing of Lazarus." (John 11:4)

Do you view yourself as worthless perhaps because you're growing older or you're retiring, and will not be productive in your usual manner? Are you appreciative of yourself as a "being" person, rather than always a human "doing"? Satan delights in accusing and/or discouraging God's people. Recognize these deceptions for the lies they are and wipe the negative ideas from your mind.

When the deceptive thoughts recur, as they probably will, fight them with the truth of Scripture: You are God's workmanship in Christ Jesus. He who began a good work in you will bring it to completion. God says, "I know the plans I have for you, plans to give you a future and a hope." Jeremiah 29:11

33. When you Question Your Relationship With God

Jesus said that He came to earth and died on a cross to make atonement for any sins you and I would ever commit - past, present, or future.

That's either true or false; you must decide what you believe.

If you accept it as true, acknowledge your sins, and ask for God's forgiveness and for strength to live without repeating sinful thoughts or actions. If you profess to be a Christian of whatever denomination, this is a truth you believe. If you're not sure, begin to talk with God, and ask him to reveal Himself and His truths to you.

Perhaps you've wished to die because you're grieving the loss of a loved one. Honestly admit and resolve your feelings about the value of your life. If necessary, seek counseling to redirect your awareness to your goodness and worth.

God loves you with an everlasting love. "The Lord hath appeared of old unto me, saying, 'Yea, I have loved thee with an everlasting love: therefore with lovingkindness have I drawn thee.'" Jeremiah 31:3

34. When You Feel Guilty

If you carry guilt for any past thoughts or actions, mentally review your transgressions during each stage of life. Write them here, and then scratch the list out with ink until it's indecipherable. Remind yourself as you flip by this page, that once you ask God's forgiveness, your sins have been forgiven and scratched out as though they never existed.

If people were harmed by your words or actions, try to privately ask their forgiveness and make amends if at all possible. If you can't reach them, confess your transgression to God, and leave it in the hands of God.

List here the items for which you wish to surrender feelings of guilt:

35. When You've Lost Hope

Wise doctors recognize that God has placed healing forces within the human body that enable it often to heal itself. Doctors do not create healing; they facilitate healing through the nature of the human body. Spontaneous remissions, totally unexplainable medically occur more often than you think.

This means even in "hopeless cases", God may miraculously intervene to create full restoration of your health. Never give up hope, unless you're peaceful and feel confident that God wants you to move into eternity. Deathbed healings have occurred.

Psalm 103:1-4 encourages your trust:

"Bless the Lord, O my soul,

And forget not all His benefits:

Who forgives all your iniquities;

Who heals all your diseases;

Who redeems your life from destruction."

Remember, nothing is impossible with God.

Meditate on the reality of this Biblical concept.

In Mark 10:27 Jesus looked at them and said, "With man this is impossible, but not with God; all things are possible with God."

36. When Your Focus Is Cloudy

Keeping a journal can help you endure difficult days more easily. And in the future, you'll be able to describe your experiences to others the better to help them. When you're finished with treatment, the journal will remind you where you've been, and give you an enriched appreciation of the future.

When you're not up to writing words in your journal, you might want to consider rating yourself on a continuum as to how well you're feeling, and how positively you're thinking. Share this with family and friends so that they may understand your daily feelings and be supportive.

FEELING: Lousy Good Great

THINKING: Lousy Good Great

37. When You Dream

Who are you, after all? What do you really like to do? Stripped of aft the "should's" from others, what are your ideal "woulds" for your life? It's time to live as you were always meant to live!

Let free-flowing dreams become your spurs to achievement in reality. Don't be a balloon bouncing here and there, but a butterfly choosing where to alight. For your greatest happiness choose your activities from the God-given desires of your heart. Don't ignore its messages. This is how God directs you into his perfect will. Examine yourself, and make plans for the future.

Desires and Dreams: I'd like to

_____

Commitment: I will

_____

In order to accomplish this, I'll take the following steps as soon as I'm able:
STEP ONE:

STEP TWO:

STEP THREE:

Share your dreams with someone who will remind you of them often.

It helps to have clear goals and written reminders for you to view often.

38. When The Day Has Ended

In the evening, when the day is done, rejoice in it. As you fall asleep at night, think about the nicest thing someone did for you that day; your favorite thought from the day; or a treasured memory you recall.

Were you able to bless someone with a kind word?

What is one joyful thought that you can anticipate the next day?

Is there someone you can pray for as you fall asleep?

"Yet the Lord will command His loving fondness in the daytime, and in the night His song shall be unto the God of your life." (Psalm 42:8)

39. When You Look Back

All that has happened to you is now part of your personal history. The events are a result of choices made by human wills, your own and those of others to whom you chose to give some power over your medical experiences. When you made your decisions you sincerely considered them the best choices at the time.

The experiences of these days can be woven by God's power and your determination into a perfect plan for your health. There have been amazing accounts of healing from every form of cancer and other serious illness.

Focus your attention on the statistics for recovery, whatever they are. Someone has to be in that number and it might as well be you. Believe in God's love and healing power, whatever you see. "And whatever things you ask in prayer, believing, you will receive." (Matt. 21:22)

40. When You Look Ahead

Yes, dream of the future. More than that, plan for it. The future is the rest of today, tomorrow, and all the tomorrows - however many. Whether sick or well, no one has a guaranteed tomorrow; in this respect, you share the uncertainty of humanity.

Go forward unafraid of the worst life has to offer, and be open to its best. Commit yourself to "go for the gold" every moment. Concentrate on making emotionally fulfilling choices in life after you've contemplated how brief human existence is. Your body is a temple of God the Holy Spirit and requires excellent care and nurturing.

"Turn away my eyes form beholding vanity; and restore me to vigorous life and health in your ways." (Psalm 119:37)

Appendix
A. Do You Need A Miraculous Healing?

Triumphing Over Cancer is designed to be used along with medical treatment. However, there are times when medicine doesn't have the answers and precise treatments you need. What then? It's important to know Jesus, the Great Healer, because it's Jesus who heals through the power of the Holy Spirit.

Jesus is waiting to give you His joy, love and healing. You can talk to Him in your heart. He's present wherever you are right now. He loves you and desires to come into your life (Revelation 3:20) according to His promise, but you must invite Him, receive Him, and believe in (Him. (John 1:12).

A simple prayer like this will do. "Jesus, thank you for dying on a cross for me. I have done and said things that I shouldn't have. I need you as my Savior and Lord. I want to follow you. Please take control of my life and make me the person you want me to be."

Does this prayer express the desire of your heart?

When you ask Jesus to heal, often He will heal you spiritually first, because there's eternal consequences of heaven or hell. (Matthew 9:1-6). Confess any sin area in your life, and get rid of bitterness or unforgiveness you have against anyone. (Mark: 24-25)

You'll realize from your study of healing verses and reading about God's goodness, love and faithfulness that Jesus still heals physically, too. Yet you must continue to ask and fill your thoughts by reading His promises in Scripture daily. (John 14:12-14). Pray believing, not doubting or despairing. (Matthew 17:14-20). Surrender the outcome totally to Him, but let there be no doubt that you've asked. It's through Jesus you were made. He can be trusted with your life.

A 25-Year Cancer Survivor's Perspective on God, Cancer & Healing
by David Rolfs

First, I believe that we must acknowledge that it is indeed God's will to heal us the moment we come before Him in prayer and claim His healing promises revealed in His word for those who are physically, mentally or spiritually sick. We need to immerse ourselves in the Biblical passages that reveal His promise to heal us, and perhaps memorize them. Surround your bed with signs that display your favorite verses. We must place our faith in what God says about illness and His desire to heal us.

We should also employ every tool for healing God has made available to us, including doctors. Surround yourself with a community of believers that will pray, fast and claim God's healing promises for you.

Network with every God-fearing church you can find, and ask to be placed on their prayer lists. Get anointed with oil by the elders of your church and ask them to pray for you on a regular basis. Visit ministers that are blessed with the gift of healing, and ask to be prayed for. Draw close to God and He will draw close to you.

Talk to God daily about your feelings concerning your illness. Try to employ humor to help you through your daily challenges. Learn as much about your illness as possible and cooperate with your doctors in your healing.

Develop an exercise program with your doctor and consult a nutritionist about making helpful dietary changes that might facilitate your body's healing process. Place all your faith in Jesus and His promises to heal you. Remember that only He can and will heal you, but act as though your healing depends on your cooperation. He gave you a mind so use it!

There are some things you should not do. Above all, do not blame yourself if you are not immediately healed, thinking you lack the faith to be healed. Remember, God does the healing and He also provides you with the faith you need to secure it if you ask Him to. Still there are times when healing is simply not God's will. His love for you is no less if this is true for you. Jesus said even a mustard seed's worth of faith could move a mountain. Leave it all up to God, after you've done your part, the rest is up to Him.

Another trap Christians often fall into is the belief that God only uses miraculous means to heal His children. Remember, there is no separation between the physical and spiritual. The Scriptures tell us that the physical world is intimately connected with the spiritual world, and that all of Creation owes its minute-to-minute existence to His sustenance. So don't think that medical healing is any less miraculous than non-medical healing.

More Thoughts About Healing

It's truly helpful if morning and evening your thoughts can be directed toward prayer and a Bible study of healing. God intends for His Word to speak to you at your point of need.

What more important topic is there for you at this time? Notice again that sometimes, although not always, God uses sickness in the way mentioned in Job 5:18. "for he wounds, but He also binds up; He injures, but His hands also heal."

Don't be afraid of God. It is never His attention to hurt you, but He may desire to nudge you and discipline you to move in a different, more wholesome direction. Sickness can be a means of motivating you.

But often the illness has nothing to do with your past behavior or choices. Don't let anyone judge you. Only God can know how He is using this. When you search your heart and seek His wisdom, He'll let you know how to respond.

As descendants of Adam, we, too, became prone to germs and genetic imperfections Adam became susceptible to when he willfully was enticed by evil. He left the perfect state in which God had made Him and made us, his descendants, vulnerable, too.

If you have any doubts about your connection to Adam genetically, read the latest genetic research on this subject that traces DNA back to one common ancestor through generations and generations. It's always helpful to meditate on the healing thoughts and verses found in Scripture.

Perhaps a family member can read them aloud to you as we used to do for our son. We also purchased recordings of healing verses to play when our son David rested. I've searched through Concordances to find the verses pertaining to Scripture that can inspire you. You may even wish to memorize your favorite verses to recite wherever you may be when you need a small jolt of encouragement.

You may want to make up your own collection of the verses most meaningful to you and record them in a special journal.

Please keep in mind the Bible is not a collection of hocus pocus words. What it is a huge compendium of truth by which we're meant to live. The more familiar you become with it, the more ingrained these thoughts will become in your mind.

Below are a few of the many verses in Scripture that pertain to heal, healed, healing, cure, cured, sick or sickness.

These verses contain the word "Healed'. Isn't it amazing there are so many references to being healed!

Genesis 20:17; 2 Chronicles 30:20; Psalm 30:2; Psalm 107:20;
    Isaiah 6:10; Isaiah 3:5; Jeremiah 17:14;
    Jeremiah 51:8 & 9; Ezekiel 34:4; Hosea 11:3;
    Matt. 4:24; Matt. 8:8; Matt. 8:13; Matt. 8:16;
    Matt. 9:21; Matt. 9:22; Matt.12:15;
    Matt. 12:22; Matt. 14:14; Matt. 14:36;
    Matt. 15:28; Matt. 15:30; Matt. 17:18; Matt. 19:2;
    Matt. 21:14; Mark 1:34; Mark 3:10; Mark 5:23;
    Mark 5:28; Mark 5:34.

There are more verses you can search out for yourself. Which healing miracle impresses you the most ?

    Mark 6:13; Mark 3:56; Mark 10:52;
    Luke 4:40; Luke 5:15; Luke 6:18; Luke 7:7;
    Luke 8:47 & 48; Luke 8:50; Luke 9:11;
    Luke 9:42; Luke 13:14; Luke 14:4;
    Luke 17:15; Luke 18:42; Luke 22:51; John 5:10;
    John 5:13; Acts 4:9 & 10; Acts 4:14;
    Acts 4:22; Acts 5:16; Acts 8:7; Acts 14:9;
    Acts 28:8; Hebrews 12:13; James 5:16; 1 Peter 2:24.

Look for the pattern in these verses of how God deals with people who ask Him for healing. Can you summarize it in a few sentences?

Checkout the word "Cure," too, in these verses:

    Luke 9:1; Matt. 8:3; Matt. 11:5; Mark 1:42; Luke 6:18;
    Luke 7:21; Luke 7:22; Luke 8:2;
    Luke 8:36; John 5:9; Acts 19:12; Acts 28:9.

Over and over Jesus cured and His followers did too. This is the Jesus you can trust.

<u>Verses with the word "Sick" also reference many healings:</u>

Proverbs 13:12; Matt. 8:16; Matt. 9:12;
Matt. 10:8; Matt. 12:15; Matt. 14:14;
Matt. 14:35 & 36; Matt. 25:39; Mark1:32;
Mark 2:17; Mark 6:5 (what a powerful thought!)
Mark 6:13; Mark 55&56; Mark16:18;
Luke 5:17; Luke 5:31; Luke 9:2; Luke 10:9;
John 4:46; John 6:2; John 11:1; John 11:2-6;
James 5:14 & 15; Acts 5:15; Acts 9:37;
Acts 19:12; Acts 28:8; Acts 28:9.
Most of these verses describe the miraculous signs Jesus performed for the sick.

<u>It's the same with verses containing the word "Sickness":</u>

Exodus 23:25; Deuteronomy 28:61; Prov. 18:14;
Jeremiah 10:19; Hosea 5:13: Matthew 4:23;
Matthew 9:35; Matthew <u>10:1; Luke 4:40; John 11:4</u>
If you ever doubt how important healing is to God, look at how many times God's involved in it!

Just as God never stopped loving the Israelites ever, even when they abused his Covenant, God never stops loving us, which is why we can approach God personally when we need healing.

Write down what you'd say to Jesus if He appeared in your room tonight?

<u>What can you learn about the kind of person God is from these verses that use the word, "Heal"?</u>

Numbers 12:13; Deut. 32:39; 2 Kings 20:5;
2 Kings 20:8; 2 Chronicles 7:14; Job 5:18;
Psalm 6:2; Psalm 41:4.

That's who God is and who are we.

A few more thoughts about these Scriptural truths:

We co-operate in our healing by the thoughts we choose to think and by the choices we make with our lives. When we live a life based on other people expectations we may not be living our own best life.

Don't you love the phrases "I'm in my glory" "I'm my best self when..." You fill in the rest – whatever delights, excites and fulfills you. Perhaps you'll say when I'm in the garden, or doing photography or putting together negotiated business deals or whatever...

We are most fully ourselves as well as emotionally healthiest when using our God-given gifts and interests. This brings life to our bones.

Share your life in community with others in some fashion. If you're an introvert you don't need to be a complete loner. Make sure you make room for people in your life. You may enjoy the social contacts you make with medical staff, simple, brief friendly conversation. You can enjoy contact with the clerk in the grocery store by asking how his or her day is going. Act as if you care about others and begin to show care and you'll be amazed at how good it makes you feel.

More verses for your meditation:
Ecclesiastes 3:3; Isaiah 19:22; Isaiah 57:18 & 19;
Jeremiah 17:14; Jeremiah 30:17;
Jeremiah 33:6; Lamentations 2:13.
Hosea 6:1; Hosea 14:4; Matt. 8:7; Matt. 10:1;
Matt. 10:8; Matt. 13:15; Mark 3:2; Mark 6:5;
Luke 5:17; Luke 7:3; Luke 8:43; Luke 9:2;
Luke 13:32; Luke 14:3; John 12:40; Acts 4:30;
Acts 28:27.

What qualities does God show in these wonderful passages of Scripture?

Have you found some favorite verses of your own as you've searched through these suggestions?

Have you written some on notecards to keep at your bedside to encourage you?

PSALM 91
FOR CANCER PATIENTS

He who dwells in the shelter of the Most High
Will abide in the shadow of the Almighty.
I will say to the Lord, My refuge and my fortress,
My God, in whom 1 trust!
For it is He who delivers you from the snare of the trapper,
And from the deadly pestilence.
He will cover you with His pinions,
And under His wings you may seek refuge;
His faithfulness is a shield and bulwark
You will not be afraid of the terror by night,
Or of the arrow that flies by day;
Of the pestilence that stalks the darkness
Or of the destruction that lays waste at noon.
A thousand may fall at your side,
And ten thousand at your right hand;
But it shall not approach you.
You will only look on with your eyes,
And see the recompense of the wielded,
For you have made the Lord, my refuge,
Even the Most High, your dwelling place.
No evil will befall you,
Nor will any plague come near your tent,
For He will give His angels charge concerning you,
To guard you in all your ways.
They will bear you up in their hands,
Lest you stride your foot against a stone,
You will tread upon the lion and cobra,
The young lion and the serpent you will trample down.
Because he has loved Me,
Therefore I will deliver him;
I will set him securely on high, because he has known My name.

He will call upon Me, and I will answer him;
I will be with him in trouble; I will rescue him, and honor him.
With a long life I will satisfy him, and let him behold My salvation."

QUESTIONS & ANSWERS ABOUT HEALING

These are some common questions patients asked by patients and caregivers during my twenty-five years of counseling patients and their families.

Why doesn't sickness disappear?

The atonement of Jesus on the cross does not mean that sickness left the earth after the Resurrection, any more than it means that sin left the earth. It does mean that we have been given grace to fight and overcome both sin and sickness. Fighting these evils is God's will.

When do you stop praying for healing?

First of all, sometimes you don't have a chance to pray before God, in His sovereignty, calls you or a loved one home through sudden sickness or an accident. But when you do have the opportunity to pray, don't give up unless your loved one is at an advanced age or God gives you peace about His taking you or your loved one into eternal life.

Not everyone is healed; we don't know why. But we're still called to pray with expectant faith. At first, our son became worse instead of better as we prayed. On the human level, it appeared as though God had abandoned us, but we refused to believe that. Continuing to trust God was not easy. It required a total commitment of our will. We often thought of Abraham walking Isaiah to the altar. He probably was hoping "Lord, surely there must be some other way." Like Abraham, we must say, "Lord we trust you, whatever."

Why aren't there more dramatic stories of miraculous healing?

Healing is often not miraculous and instantaneous. More often God uses a process of healing over a period of time, thereby touching many more lives. God uses all things, even evil, for good - transforming and perfecting his children in the process.

Is trust something I either have or don't have or something I can acquire?

Webster defines trust as assured reliance on the character, ability, strength, or truth of someone or something; complete confidence. Trust seems to be like an action. Ex. Prov. 3:5 'Trust in the Lord with all thy heart." I Chron. 5:20 "...for they cried out to God in the battle. He heeded their prayer, because they put their trust in Him." God respects trust.

Is trusting in God's healing power all that I need to do?

Jesus used natural and supernatural means to perform his acts of healing. He rubbed the blind man's eyes with mud, remember, and said 'The well have no need of a physician, only the sick." We can conclude that He believed the sick did need to use doctors. You and your loved ones need to take an active part medically, too. That involves more than simply passive trusting. During our son's fight with cancer we all prayed for wisdom and were actively involved in gathering the knowledge needed to make sound medical decisions for David."In all things give thanks..." is the correct Christian concept along with "Having done all, stand." We are to take an active role working for the restoration of our health when we're sick.

What is the Scriptural foundation for healing?

The Scriptural foundation for healing is found in Isaiah 53 which states that at the time of the Atonement, when Jesus died on the cross, He took upon Himself our sins and "...by His stripes, we are healed." The words of Matthew confirm this in Matthew 8: 17 which quotes Isaiah: "...and all the sick were healed." This fulfilled the prophecy of Isaiah. "He took our sicknesses and bore our diseases.

What if healing is not God's will?

Too often Christians take the wishy-washy attitude that's reflected in the prayer: "Lord, if it be thy will, please heal me." There is NO biblical foundation for timid prayer or thoughts like this. There is biblical foundation for expectant prayer and for action toward healing. When asked to heal, Jesus never said first, I must go pray if it's God's will that I heal you. He knew His Father's love and power.

Isn't there a value in suffering?

Yes, there can be. But that is not always God's plan. If it were, why did Jesus heal anyone? Examine these foundational facts. Suffering is certainly part of life in this world. Suffering is sometimes used by Him to wake people up to spiritual realities that they have been missing. Sometimes the person who suffers has not been afflicted for his own sins but only to influence certain other individuals. Perhaps his sickness is simply a display arena for God's power.

<u>Is God's willingness to heal dependent upon someone's worthiness?</u>

When Jesus walked this earth, He healed all who asked. He heard the prayer of the centurion, "Lord 1 am not worthy, but only say the word, and he shall be healed." We do not merit healing any more than we merit salvation.

<u>What if I've waited too long and my sickness is too advanced?</u>

You know the answer to that. God is a God of the impossible. The Christian need not be daunted by medical opinion regarding the impossibility of healing. Abraham and Sarah would undoubtedly have failed all medical fertility tests at their advanced ages; yet God saw fit to confound obvious physical factors. No matter what your medical prognosis God can heal you. You are called to have faith.

<u>What's the people's response to Jesus' healing power today?</u>

Matt. 9: 1-8. When the people brought Jesus a paralyzed man on a bed, Jesus seeing their faith said. Be of good cheer, thy sins are forgiven. The Pharisees questioned Jesus' ability to forgive sins. Today we do not question Jesus' willingness to forgive all sins, but some question His willingness to heal sickness.

<u>Why would God want to heal us?</u>

Is He any less loving than an earthly father who cannot bear to see his child in pain? Does He not love us today as much as He loved people in the past? Has He failed to make provision for us? What kind of Father would leave His children to suffer if he had the means to alleviate it?

<u>How did Jesus confirm His ability to forgive sins?</u>

"But that you may know that the Son of man hath power on earth to forgive sins, he said to the sick man, Arise, take up your bed and walk."

<u>How can I facilitate my own healing?</u>

Soak yourself in the knowledge of God's words on His love and healing.
Read the testimony of those who have been miraculously healed.
Surround yourself with a community of people who have faith in healing.

A Special Note to Caregivers

I know it's scary. All the things you wanted to do for your loved one,

The I-should have's and the I- didn'ts pass through your mind.

You want to clutch the person you care about and say, "you can't go, you can't leave me."

Then later you catch yourself trying to envision how you might make it through life alone.

You feel guilty and tell your brain to stop, my loved one will live!

Oh, it can be such a wild, confusing time.

You give and give and become exhausted.

You know you need rest and you try, but it's not easy to find a competent replacement.

Plus you just want to be with your dear one as much as you can.

Then even when you have a break from the physical strain,

The mental remains and it's just as horrid.

Don't be frightened. Turn to God. He's your deep and real comfort.

Ask Him each day to show you through His Spirit how you can best help your loved one.

Read these ideas carefully.

Then follow the suggestions that seem right for you and your beloved.

May God bless and guide you and help you and your loved *one through this.*

ACKNOWLEDGMENTS

MANY THANKS TO THE NURSING STAFF AT UNIVERSITY-WISCONSIN MADISON, DR. HONG, DR. LOVE, DR. ERSHLER, DR. BLOCK, DR. KNAVEL, PASTORS WINKLER AND DAVID HAWLEY AND FATHER JIM VOJTIK, THE CURSILLO COMMUNITY OF DELAVAN, MILWAUKEE AND RACINE AND THE PRAYER COMMUNITIES ACROSS THE UNITED STATES AND IN THE CAYMAN ISLANDS.

ABOUT THE AUTHOR

Dr. Judith Rolfs cares passionately about God and families. She's been a professional marriage and family counselor for over twenty-five years. Because of her personal experience with her teen-age son's cancer she has a special concern for patients and families fighting the emotional and physical devastation of cancer or any life-threatening illness.

Dr. Rolfs has done extensive research on the emotional and spiritual components of cancer treatment, particularly in the field of psychoneuroimmunology. Her books have been distributed worldwide as tools to help others through the maze of cancer treatment.

OTHER BOOKS BY DR. JUDITH ROLFS:

Never Tomorrow, inspirational adult mystery novel

Directive 99, adult suspense novel

Bullet In The Night, mystery novel set in Lake Geneva, WI

52 Ways To Keep Your Promises As A Husband and Father

Man in Command, How To Be A Great Dad and Husband

Loving Every Minute, 52 Ways To Live, Laugh & Love

Breathless Devotional Mini-Meditations

God Thoughts, Devotions For Every Day

Love Notes To God, 365-Day Devotionals

Soaring As A Parent, Secrets To Being Great

Secrets To Being A Super Grandparent

For Children:

Tommy Smurlee and Dunster's Camp of Mystery & Inventions

Tommy Smurlee and the Missing Statue

Hey, I've Got ADHD, Here's How You Can Help

Hey, I've Got Cancer, Here's How You Can Help

Truth for Teens, Answers to Life's Tough Questions

Unforgettable Stories For Kids

All books are available at amazon.com

If you found the material in *Triumphing Over Cancer* helpful please encourage others to read it by leaving a review on the book's page on Amazon.

Visit Dr. Judith Rolfs' Website

www.judithrolfs.com